first place
4health

Bible Study Series

celebrate
success

Published by Gospel Light
Ventura, California, U.S.A.
www.gospellight.com
Printed in the U.S.A.

Caution: The information contained in this book is intended to be solely for
informational and educational purposes. It is assumed that the First Place 4 Health
participant will consult a medical or health professional before beginning this or
any other weight-loss or physical fitness program.

Library of Congress Cataloging-in-Publication Data
Celebrate success.
p. cm. — (First place 4 health bible study series)
Includes bibliographical references and index.
ISBN 978-0-8307-4755-9 (trade paper : alk. paper)
1. Spiritual life—Christianity—Study and teaching.
I. Gospel Light Publications (Firm)
BV4511.C44 2009
242'.5—dc22
2008056110

Rights for publishing this book outside the U.S.A. or in non-English
languages are administered by Gospel Light Worldwide, an international
not-for-profit ministry. For additional information, please visit
www.glww.org, email info@glww.org, or write to Gospel Light Worldwide,
1957 Eastman Avenue, Ventura, CA 93003, U.S.A.

contents

foreword

My introduction to Bible study came when I joined First Place in March 1981. I had been attending church since I was a small child, but the extent of my study of the Bible had been reading my Sunday School quarterly on Saturday night. On Sunday morning, I would listen to my Sunday School teacher as she taught God's Word to me. During the worship service, I would listen to our pastor as he taught God's Word to me. Frankly, digging out the truths of the Bible for myself had never entered my mind.

Perhaps you are right where I was back in 1981. If so, you are in for a blessing you never dreamed possible. As you start studying the truths of the Bible for yourself through the First Place 4 Health Bible studies, you will see God begin to open your understanding of His Word.

Almost every First Place 4 Health member I have talked with about the program says, "The weight loss is wonderful, but the most important thing I have received from my association with First Place 4 Health is learning to study God's Word." The First Place 4 Health Bible studies are designed to be done on a daily basis. As you work through each day's study (which will take 15 to 20 minutes to complete), you will be discovering the deep truths of God's Word. A part of each week's study will also include a Bible memory verse for the week.

There are many in-depth Bible studies on the market. The First Place 4 Health Bible studies are not designed for the purpose of in-depth study, but are designed to be used in conjunction with the rest of the program to bring balance into your life. Our desire is for each member to begin having a personal quiet time with God each day. This time alone with God should include a time of prayer, Bible reading and Bible study. Having a quiet time is a daily discipline that will bring the rich rewards of balance, which is something we all need.

God bless you as you begin this exciting journey toward a balanced life. God will richly bless your efforts to give Him first place in your life. Remember Matthew 6:33: "But seek first his kingdom and his righteousness, and all these things will be given to you as well."

Carole Lewis, First Place 4 Health National Director

introduction

First Place 4 Health is a Christ-centered health program that emphasizes balance in the physical, mental, emotional and spiritual areas of life. The First Place 4 Health program is meant to be a daily process. As we learn to keep Christ first in our lives, we will find that He is the One who satisfies our hunger and our every need.

This Bible study is designed to be used in conjunction with the First Place 4 Health program but can be beneficial for anyone interested in obtaining a balanced lifestyle. The Bible study has been created in a five-day format, with the last two days reserved for reflection on the material studied. Keep in mind that the ultimate goal of studying the Bible is not only for knowledge but also for application and a changed life. Don't feel anxious if you can't seem to find the *correct* answer. Many times, the Word will speak differently to different people, depending on where they are in their walk with God and the season of life they are experiencing.

There are some other components included with this study that help you as you pursue the goal of giving Christ first place in your life:

- **Group Prayer Request Form:** This form is at the end of each week's study. You can use this to record any special requests that might be given in class.

- **Leader Discussion Guide:** This discussion guide is provided to help the First Place 4 Health leader guide a group through this Bible study. It includes ideas for facilitating a First Place 4 Health class discussion for each week of the Bible study.

- **Two Weeks of Menu Plans with Recipes:** There are 14 days of meals, and all are interchangeable. Each day totals 1,400 to 1,500 calories and includes snacks. An accompanying grocery list includes items that will be needed for each week of meals.

- **First Place 4 Health Member Survey:** Fill this out and bring it to your first meeting. This information will help your leader know your interests and talents.

- **Personal Weight and Measurement Record:** Use this form to keep a record of your weight loss. Record any loss or gain on the chart after the weigh-in at each week's meeting.

- **Weekly Prayer Partner Forms:** Fill out this form before class and place it into a basket during the class meeting. After class, you will draw out a prayer request form, and this will be your prayer partner for the week. Try to call or email the person sometime before the next class meeting to encourage that person.

- **Live It Trackers:** Your Live It Tracker is to be completed at home and turned in to your leader at your weekly First Place 4 Health meeting. The Tracker is designed to help you practice mindfulness and stay accountable with regard to your eating and exercise habits. Step-by-step instructions for how to use the Live It Tracker are provided in the *Member's Guide*.

- **Let's Count Our Miles!** A worthy goal we encourage is for you to complete 100 miles of exercise during your 12 weeks in First Place 4 Health. There are many activities listed on pages 255-256 that count toward your goal of 100 miles. When you complete a mile of activity, mark off the box listed on the Hundred Mile Club chart located on the inside of the back cover.

- **Scripture Memory Cards:** These cards have been designed so you can use them while exercising. It is suggested that you punch a hole in the upper left corner and place the cards on a ring. You may want to take the cards in the car or to work so you can practice each week's Scripture memory verse throughout the day.

- **Scripture Memory CD:** All 10 Scripture memory verses have been put to music at an exercise tempo in the CD at the back of this study. Use this CD when exercising or even when you are just driving in your car. The words of Scripture are often easier to memorize when accompanied by music.

Use each of these important tools found in this study to live a balanced and healthy life.

welcome to
Celebrate Success

At your first group meeting for this session of First Place 4 Health, you will meet your fellow members, get an overview of your materials and find out what you can expect at weekly meetings. The majority of your class time will be spent learning about the four-sided person concept, the Live It Food Plan, and how change begins from the inside out. You will also have a chance to ask any questions about how to get the most out of First Place 4 Health. If possible, complete the Member Survey on page 205 before your first group meeting. The information that you give will help your leader tailor the next 12 weeks to the needs of the whole group.

Each weekly meeting begins with a weigh-in for members. This will allow you to track your progress over the 12-week session. Your Week One weigh-in/measurement will establish a baseline of comparison so that you can set healthy goals for this session. If you are apprehensive about weighing in every week, talk with your group leader about your concerns. He or she will have some options for you to consider that will make the weigh-in activity encouraging rather than stressful.

The day after your first meeting, begin Week Two of this Bible study. This session, you and your group will learn to make wise choices that lead to celebrating success in First Place 4 Health, even as you learn what celebration looks like in the kingdom of God. As you open yourself to the truth of Scripture and share your hopes and struggles with the members of your group during the next 12 weeks, you'll find yourself becoming the healthy child of God you are designed to be!

celebrate love and faithfulness

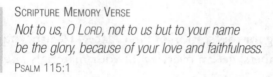

*Not to us, O LORD, not to us but to your name
be the glory, because of your love and faithfulness.*
PSALM 115:1

"Celebrate success." Just saying those words can bring joy to your heart and mind and put a smile on your face. Pause for a moment and say those words out loud: "celebrate success." What mental pictures and emotions does that phrase bring up for you? Describe those feelings and images in the space below.

_____

_____

_____

_____

All too often, we think of celebrating success as something to do when we have finally attained a long-awaited goal or received special recognition or reached a milestone in life. However, for those who strive to live a life pleasing to God, celebrating success can be a daily experience, not just an isolated event. Each evening before you go to bed, you can hear the Lord saying to you, "Well done, good and faithful servant! You have been faithful with a few things; I will put you in charge of many things. Come and share your master's happiness!" (Matthew 25:21).

Just as you did with the phrase "celebrate success," read the words of Matthew 25:21 out loud. Let the emotions associated with Jesus' words well up inside you. Now describe the feelings and images this verse brings up for you.

How were these images and feelings the same as what the words "celebrate success" evoked in you? How were they different? Often, we miss the joy of our Master's happiness because we try to measure success by the world's yardstick—and tape measure—rather than allowing God to define what success looks like in the lives of His disciples.

CALLED AND ENTRUSTED

Day 1

Gracious God, You have entrusted me with the awesome responsibility of caring for myself because of Your great care for me. Help me today, and always, to be faithful in this one thing. Amen.

In the parable of the talents, Jesus helps us understand what success looks like in the kingdom of God. As we begin our *Celebrate Success* journey, let's turn our eyes toward Jesus and the words He used to enable us to better understand what success looks like when pictured through God's eyes.

Turn to Matthew 25:14-23 and read the first segment of this parable of the talents. As you read Jesus' words, keep in mind that He told parables as a means of describing more abstract concepts to His listeners. By using concrete examples that they could easily relate to and understand, Jesus could explain a complex spiritual concept that their finite minds would have otherwise had a difficult time grasping.

In order to understand the "it" referred to in Matthew 25:14, look at the beginning of Matthew 25 and read verse 1. Based on this, what does the "it" in Matthew 25:14 refer to?

_____

_____

_____

In this passage, Jesus is using another story-type example to help His listeners understand what the kingdom of heaven will be like. What is that example?

_____

_____

_____

According to Matthew 25:14, what did the man going on a journey do?

_____

_____

_____

Place a bookmark in the Matthew 25 passage and then turn to John 16:5. After reading John 16:5, who is the man spoken of in Matthew 25:14 who is going away on a journey?

_____

_____

_____

Jesus is going back to the One who sent Him and, like the man in the parable, He is calling His disciples and entrusting His property to them. According to Matthew 8:20, what kind of property did Jesus have to entrust to His followers?

_____

_____

_____

We know from Scripture that Jesus' kingdom was not an earthly kingdom and that Jesus did not have physical property to leave to His disciples. Based on your reading of this parable, what is one of the "talents" Jesus has entrusted to you, His modern-day disciple?

_____

_____

_____

_____

What are you doing in your life right now that is helping you to be a wise and prudent steward of the things that God has given you?

_____

_____

_____

_____

Thank You, Lord God Almighty, for calling me to be a wise and prudent steward of all You have given me, beginning with the care and maintenance of my relationship with You. Amen.

ACCORDING TO OUR ABILITY

Day 2

O Lord God, what You are asking of me is not beyond my reach. Help me to be faithful according to the ability You have given me. Amen.

Yesterday's lesson introduced a teaching found in Matthew 25:14-23. Reread this passage as you begin today's lesson. What new information did the Holy Spirit illuminate for you in today's reading—something that was hidden from your spiritual eyes yesterday?

_____

_____

_____

_____

Yesterday, we looked at a parable of a man who was going away on a journey. Again, who is the man being spoken of in Matthew 25:14, and who are the servants he called and entrusted with his property?

_____

_____

_____

_____

You also discovered yesterday that the care of your physical body is one of the "talents" Jesus has entrusted to you. Yet in Matthew 25:14, we are told the man entrusted "his" property to the servants. How is your body part of Jesus' property? (Read 1 Corinthians 3:16 and 6:19-20 before answering this question.)

_____

_____

_____

_____

First Corinthians 6:20 tells us that we were bought at a price. What was the price? (See 1 Peter 1:18-19 for help to answer this question.)

_____

_____

_____

_____

Going back to the parable of the talents, we glean another piece of valuable information in Matthew 25:15. What are we told about the distribution of the talents?

_____

_____

_____

_____

Who was the one who decided who got what? On what criteria was this decision based?

_____

_____

_____

_____

_____

What does this passage tell you about comparing yourself to others in your First Place 4 Health group, or in your church, or in another circle of friends?

_____

_____

_____

_____

_____

_____

When we compare ourselves to others and allow ourselves to feel as though we have not been given as much ability as they have been given, who are we really criticizing?

_____

_____

_____

_____

End your study time today by thanking God for entrusting you with the things He knows you have the ability to achieve—these things are not too difficult for you or beyond your reach!

> O loving and merciful God, You created me, and You care for me.
> Today, I ask that You empower me to care for myself in a way that
> brings glory and honor to You, my Creator. Amen.

Day 3 ENTRUSTED AND ACCOUNTABLE

*My faithful Father, You made me and You sustain me. How grateful
I am for Your presence in my life. How thankful I am that I can share in
Your joy as I take care of myself in a way that honors You. Amen.*

In the parable of the talents, Jesus teaches that talents are given to His
servants according to His knowledge of their ability (see Matthew
25:15). How does Psalm 139:1-4 and 13-16 affirm this truth?

_____

_____

_____

What does Psalm 139:14 say that we are to do in response to our being
created by God?

_____

_____

_____

Psalm 139:14 declares that we are "fearfully and wonderfully made."
Obviously, this is not the frightened type of fear that goes hand in hand
with worry and anxiety. Look up the word "fear" in a dictionary and see
if you can find an alternate definition that better explains what the
psalmist is saying in this verse.

_____

_____

_____

_____

How is frightened fear different from the reverential awe we are called
to consider when we think of the way God created our physical being?

_____

_____

_____

Unlike people who have much according to the world's power structure, those who have been given much in God's kingdom do not have special rank and privilege or a reason to lord it over others. What does the second half of Luke 12:48 tell us about those who have been given much?

_____

_____

_____

_____

Turn to 1 Corinthians 4:2. What does the apostle Paul tell us we are to do with those things with which we have been entrusted?

_____

_____

_____

_____

How might the phrase "faithful with a few things" in Matthew 25:21 help you understand the truth that Jesus is teaching in this parable? (Consider how a "few things" differ from "all things" as you answer this question.)

_____

_____

_____

_____

_____

What are the "few things" we have been entrusted with, and how might trying to do "all things" keep us from doing the few things Jesus has entrusted to our care?

_____

_____

_____

_____

_____

What does this teach you about the importance of right priorities?

_____

_____

_____

_____

What is one thing relating to your First Place 4 Health journey in which you have proven faithful today?

_____

_____

_____

_____

Celebrate your success by praising the God who entrusts and empowers you to do His will!

Lord God, forgive me for the times I get so wrapped up in doing "all things" that I neglect the "few things" You ask of me. Gracious God, teach me to order my priorities in a way that pleases You. Amen.

Day 4

WHO GETS THE CREDIT?

Lord, thank You for all of the gifts that You have entrusted to my care. Help me to be a good steward of all that You have given to me. Amen.

This week's memory verse adds yet another dimension to the parable of the talents. We are the servants who are called and entrusted, yet even as we are faithful in a few things, we cannot claim any of the credit for our accomplishments! Write out this week's memory verse below. Circle who gets the credit, and then underline why credit is due this person.

_____

_____

_____

Based on Matthew 25:14-15, why is God the one who gets the glory, even though we have done the work?

_____

_____

_____

_____

The Lord is the one who gives us the talents! They are His possessions, committed to our safekeeping. But there is more—much more. Without God's love and faithfulness, there is simply no way we could use these talents for God's glory. Jesus explained this truth in John 15:4. Read that verse, and then explain in your own words what Jesus is saying.

_____

_____

_____

_____

On the left-hand side of the following three-column chart are a few verses that speak of God's love and faithfulness. After reading each of the passages, list the aspect of God's faithfulness being addressed in those verses in the center column. Then, in the right-hand column, write how this aspect of God's faithfulness allows you to be a faithful steward of the good things entrusted to your care.

Verse	Aspect of God's love/faithfulness described in this verse	How God's faithfulness and love allow me to be a good steward
Ps. 86:15		
Ps. 91:3-4		
Ps. 94:18		

Verse	Aspect of God's love/faithfulness described in this verse	How God's faithfulness and love allow me to be a good steward
Lam. 3:22-23		
1 Cor. 10:13		
1 Thess. 5:23-24		
Heb. 10:22-23		

Spend the rest of your study time praising and thanking God for His love and faithfulness.

Mighty and sovereign Lord, You are the one who deserves all the glory and honor and praise. You are loving and faithful. Without Your love and faithfulness, I could do no good thing! Amen.

Day
5

THE IMPORTANCE OF KNOWING GOD

Merciful Lord, You call me into relationship and invite me to learn about You. In Your Word, You reveal Yourself to me. Help me read Your Word and meditate on Your goodness and grace today and always. Amen.

There is one other servant in the parable of the talents, and he, too, has a valuable lesson to teach us. Turn in your Bible to Matthew 25 and read verses 24-30. The two servants described in Matthew 25:14-23 managed their talents to the best of their ability, and because they were "faithful in little," they were given more—and invited to share in their master's happiness. But Jesus tells us that the third servant was not faithful.

What did the third servant do, and what was the end result?

_____

_____

_____

_____

At first glance, it is easy to think that the master is treating this servant harshly; after all, the servant was afraid. Yet when we read the truth of Jesus' words, we quickly see this servant through new eyes. In Matthew 25:24-30, we discover the root of the problem. What was the source of this man's fear and, consequently, his failure to act responsibly?

_____

_____

_____

_____

_____

In Matthew 25:26, Jesus calls the servant _____ and _____. Even though this man was a servant, he had not learned the truth about his master's attributes and character. He did not understand his master's plan and purpose. He did not take the time to get to know the master intimately.

In his letter to the Ephesians, the apostle Paul prays that the Ephesian Christians will be "rooted and established in love" (Ephesians 3:17). Read Paul's entire prayer recorded in Ephesians 3:14-21. Summarize what Paul is saying about knowing the height and breadth, depth and width of God's love and what this knowledge does for you.

_____

_____

_____

_____

_____

What have you learned about God's love and faithfulness in this week's lesson that you did not know before?

_____

_____

_____

_____

Learning more about God is always a reason to celebrate success! Each and every day, you can get to know God at a deeper level as you read and meditate on His Word and talk to Him. Truly, we serve a God of compassion, mercy and love!

> *O Lord God, to the faithful You show Yourself faithful; to the blameless You show Yourself blameless. You, O Lord, are the one who keeps my lamp burning and turns my darkness into light (see Psalm 18:25-28). Amen.*

Day
6

REFLECTION AND APPLICATION

Lord God, You invite me into an intimate, interactive love relationship with You. Although it is too much for my finite mind to grasp, I am grateful for Your faithfulness and love—and for the invitation to get to know You as intimately as You know me! Amen.

During the Day Four study this week, you looked at several aspects of God's faithfulness and then considered how that aspect of His character allowed you to be a faithful steward. Go back to that lesson and review your work. As you read over the list, ask the Holy Spirit to illuminate the aspect of God's faithfulness that you need to experience at a deeper level of your being so that you can be more faithful in your service to Him.

When the Holy Spirit has given you insight, list that aspect of God's faithfulness below and spend some time talking to God in prayer, asking Him to reveal Himself to you in new and exciting ways. Talk to God about the misconceptions that you might have had that have kept you from claiming His promises, accepting His forgiveness, or believing that He is your shield in times of trouble and your deliverer when you are tempted. (You might want to complete this exercise in your prayer journal.) End your prayer time by thanking God in advance for proving Himself faithful and loving in response to your prayer.

The aspect of God's faithfulness that I need to experience at a deeper level today is:

_____

_____

_____

_____

At the end of the *Celebrate Success* Bible study, you will be asked to list the ways in which God has shown Himself faithful to you in this area. You can be sure there will be many! Our God is a God who delights in revealing Himself to His faithful servants.

> *Thank You, gracious Lord, for revealing Yourself to me in new and exciting ways as I read and meditate on Your Word. Thank You for loving me enough to send Jesus to die for me so that I can be in a right relationship with You. Amen.*

REFLECTION AND APPLICATION Day 7

Praise the Lord, O my soul; all my inmost being, praise his holy name. Praise the Lord, O my soul, and forget not all his benefits—who forgives all your sins and heals all your diseases (see Psalm 103:1-2).

In Psalm 103:3-5, David lists six specific benefits he derived from God's faithfulness and love. Those six benefits are listed on the following chart. Next to each benefit, describe how God's faithfulness in this area has helped you in your journey to put Christ first in all things in your life. (If you have not experienced this aspect of God's faithfulness, ask the Lord, by the power of His Holy Spirit, to apply this benefit to your heart and mind in new and exciting ways.)

Benefit	How I have experienced this benefit because of God's love and faithfulness
He crowns me with love and compassion	
He satisfies my desires with good things	
He renews my youth like the eagle's	
He forgives all my sins	
He heals all my diseases	
He redeems me from the pit	

Spend some time praising God and meditating on all His benefits in your life!

Lord God, You are compassionate and gracious, slow to anger, abounding in love. Thank You that my soul can praise You, for You have been good to me! Amen.

Group Prayer Requests

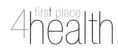

Today's Date: _____

Name	Request

Results

_____

_____

_____

_____

_____

_____

celebrate hope for a better tomorrow

SCRIPTURE MEMORY VERSE
Praise be to the God and Father of our Lord Jesus Christ!
In his great mercy he has given us new birth into a living hope
through the resurrection of Jesus Christ from the dead.
1 PETER 1:3

It is fitting to celebrate when you have accomplished something pleasing to God. And when you have done what is pleasing to the Lord, not only do you celebrate, but God also celebrates with you!

Last week we considered our Lord's words, "Well done, good and faithful servant! You have been faithful with a few things; I will put you in charge of many things. Come and share your master's happiness!" (Matthew 25:23). Recall what feelings and mental pictures those words brought up for you.

Did you have occasion to hear those words during the week as you were faithful to care for the body God has given you to carry out His work in the world? If so, briefly describe what your faithfulness looked like.

_____

_____

_____

_____

_____

The prophet Zephaniah gives us another visual image of what it means to celebrate in the kingdom of God. Turn to Zephaniah 3:17 and write what God is doing in that passage.

He will take great delight in you
He will quiet you
He will rejoice over you

What images and feelings does the truth that God rejoices over you with singing bring up for you?

He is satisfied with my work

In order to celebrate success, we must first be willing to pay the price that success requires. We must be willing to hold on to visions of celebrating success even during times when we are struggling to just put one foot in front of the other or when we feel that in spite of our best efforts we are losing ground. Success is defined by faithfulness over a period of time and is not always easily acquired.

CONSIDER THE COST

Day 1

Lord, thank You for reminding me of the need to plan and prepare before I begin rebuilding my life according to Your specifications. Amen.

While the world promotes the thrill of celebration in order to motivate us to action, Jesus invites us to consider something else: the cost of commitment. Even as our Savior invited men and women to follow Him, He never painted a picture of "no cost" celebration!

To illustrate the need to consider the cost, Jesus gave the large crowds who were traveling with Him an example to help them better understand this particular Kingdom principle. Turn in your Bible to Luke 14:28-30 and read that example. What does the person in this story aspire to do (see v. 28)?

build a tower

What does Jesus say the person who desires to build a tower must first do (see v. 28)?

estimate the cost

What does Jesus say will happen if the person lays the foundation and is not able to finish the project (see v. 29)?

everyone will ridicule him

When we begin a self-improvement project without first considering the cost, our plans and dreams will not result in permanent change. How can considering the cost of a plan help ensure our success?

we must to the cost in order to carry out our plans

What are some of the costs you must consider when seeking to live a healthy life? (Include costs like time and energy as well as the cost of doing things differently from the way you have done them in the past. Change requires energy and effort!)

Am I willing to spend the time & energy to change my life. must plan on my budget if I can buy the right food

As you conclude today's study, think about whether these are costs that you are truly willing to pay and talk to God about your willingness to pay this price for success. (You might want to record your conversation in the pages of your prayer journal.)

> *Gracious God, how often I want instant transformation when the reality is that in Your kingdom, considering the cost is the pathway to success. Today, I want to consider the cost of doing the things that are pleasing to You. Thank You, Lord. Amen.*

THE TENT OF MEETING
Day 2

> *Gracious and loving Lord, so often I want to serve two masters; to be at peace with You as well as enjoy the success offered by the world. You tell me that I must choose between whom I will serve. Today, I choose You. Amen.*

In yesterday's lesson, you examined the cost of building a tower. Recall one of the building costs you were willing to pay in order to glorify God with your body and write that below.

time spend with God

Having considered the cost, what plans have you made to make this dream a reality?

I must have a different mind set

Proverbs 16:3 tells us that there is something else we must be willing to do in addition to considering the cost. What is the wisdom contained in this verse, and how is this essential step also a cost (albeit a hidden one) of success?

time spent with the Lord

In order to commit our plans to the Lord, we must first know what God wants us to do. What are you doing to better understand what God desires of you? What is the cost involved?

In order to understand what God desires of us, we must be willing to read and meditate on His Word. We must spend quality time with Him, seeking His will and listening to His voice. Turn in your Bible to Exodus 33:7-11. This passage tells something very specific that Moses did with a tent. What does the first sentence in Exodus 33:7 tell you?

He was preparing a place for a meeting with God

Notice that Moses set up this structure outside the camp, some distance away. Why was it essential that it be outside the camp?

So that people had to want to come to the meeting place

Are you willing to pay the cost of separating yourself from the busyness of your world so you can meet with the Lord each day? Why or why not?

Yes

Those who are serious about their relationship with the Lord have a special place to meet with God each day; their own "tent of meeting," so to speak. Describe your tent of meeting and the things you take into your tent when you go to speak to the Lord face to face.

Spend the rest of your quiet time today thanking God that He has called you into an intimate relationship with Him and that He invites you to commit your plans to Him so that they will succeed.

Thank You, loving Lord, for meeting with me each day and showing me the path You would have me take. Having committed my plans to You, I will go out into the world, confident that they will succeed.

Day 3

OTHERS WATCH US WORSHIP

Almighty and merciful God, it is often difficult for me to make time in my busy day to step away and spend time with You. Help me to be faithful and always willing to commit my plans to You. Thank You. Amen.

During yesterday's lesson, you read about the tent of meeting. Exodus 33:7 ends with this sentence: "Anyone inquiring of the LORD would go to the tent of meeting outside the camp." What did you learn yesterday about the importance of going to the tent of meeting, and why was it necessary that this tent be pitched outside the camp?

it is important to sometimes be alone with our talk to Jesus

Exodus 33:8 tells us that something else happened whenever Moses went out to the tent. What was this?

the other people stood at the entrance to their tent watching Moses

When we are willing to separate ourselves and inquire of the Lord, others observe our actions! How could allowing others to witness our commitment to spend quality time with God be considered another "cost" of success?

we must always be faithful to our talk to Jesus.

What does Exodus 33:10 say the people did when they saw Moses meeting with God?

they stood & worshiped

How might your willingness to come apart each day and spend time meeting with God encourage others to worship?

They can see that we are happy with our commitment to Jesus

What does Exodus 33:9 say happened when Moses went inside the tent of meeting?

a cloud would come down & stay at the entrance.

What might this tell you about how important it is to God that you spend dedicated time with Him?

He wants us one on one as well as in a group

God desires that we spend time with Him—time that is free from outside distractions. How is this truth reinforced by Psalm 139:5-6?

He hems us in so we can be alone with Him

Based on everything you have read in this passage, why is it so important for us to not allow other commitments and obligations to interfere with our appointment with God each day?

He wants to meet with us & we should want to meet with Him

How is spending time each day with God the most effective type of personal evangelism that you can possibly engage in—beneficial to you and to those who watch you worship?

we all gain from time spent with God

_____

_____

_____

_____

> *Gracious God, thank You for hemming me in behind and before so that I can have quiet, uninterrupted time with You. Thank You that this time spent apart with You can be a powerful witness to others. Amen.*

Day 4

FACE TO FACE

> *Loving and merciful Lord, it is beyond my ability to comprehend the truth that the God of heaven and earth would want to spend time with me! Thank You for inviting me into Your presence. Amen.*

This week, you have been looking at the importance of considering the cost of success as a prelude to celebrating success. You have looked at many different types of costs that are involved in achieving success. List one cost that you had not previously considered as a factor in your commitment to give Christ first place in your life. Then list what you are going to do to "pay" that price.

Cost factor: _____

_____

_____

What I will do to pay the price: _____

_____

_____

As a result of Moses' willingness to pitch a tent of meeting and faithfully go to that meeting place each day, he was able to celebrate success. According to Exodus 33:11, what was that success?

The _Lord_ would _speak_ to _Moses_ _face_ to _face_, as a man _speaks_ with his _friend_.

What is so amazing about this verse when you consider who God is and who we are?

that God would come to the lowly ones.

How is it a reason to celebrate?

God loves each of us.

Is this a type of success that the world understands or values? Why or why not?

everyone wants to think they are better than some others

Turn in your Bible to Jeremiah 9:23-24. What do these verses tell you about the importance of your relationship with the Lord?

We must know God & boast about Him & things He has done

Jeremiah 9:23 lists three things our society boasts about—and considers grounds for celebration. What are those three things?

1. _boast of wisdom_
2. _boast of strength_
3. _boast of riches_

Look over the list you just made. Are those things acquired instantly, or is there a cost involved in acquiring them? Explain your answer.

these things do not come easily

The Lord, through Jeremiah, tells us that His value system is different from the things valued by the world. What does Jeremiah 9:24 say is important to the Lord?

that we boast about knowing God we know He exercises kindness, justice, righteousness on earth. for in these God delight

How is understanding and knowing the Lord a reason for celebration? How does this truth correspond to what you learned in your study of Exodus 33:7-11?

because we become close to Him & know Him as a friend

Thank You, loving Lord, for showing me the difference between the things that delight You and the things the world delights in. Help me always to strive to know and understand You and to spend time in Your presence learning about You. Amen.

CELEBRATING CHRIST'S RESURRECTION

*My Lord and my God, I often am so busy celebrating temporal things
that I forget to celebrate the most important event in human history:
Your resurrection! Help me, Lord, to celebrate my new hope in You.*

Each Easter, Christians throughout the world gather to celebrate the
most important event in history. Write this week's memory verse below,
and then circle the event and underline the benefit we receive because
Jesus Christ was willing to pay the price of our salvation.

*Praise be to God and Father of our Lord Jesus
Christ. In his great mercy he has given us
new birth into a living hope through the resurrection
of Jesus Christ from the dead. 1 Peter 1:3*

Hebrews 12:2-3 gives us a vivid description of the price Jesus was willing to pay so that we could have new birth and a living hope. Read this
passage and then describe in your own words the price that Jesus paid.

*Jesus suffered sever pain & died on the
cross, so that we could be forgiven of
our sins*

The apostle Paul calls the benefits we receive from Christ's willingness
to pay the cost "spiritual blessings" (see Ephesians 1:3). In that verse,
Paul says that we have been blessed with "every spiritual blessing." What
are some of the spiritual blessings you have received because Jesus Christ
died and was raised to new life on the third day? (You might want to
read Ephesians 1:4-8 as you formulate your list.)

We were chosen before the creation of the world to be holy and blameless in God's sight. To be "holy" is to be set apart; to be separate. How is spending time alone with God each day part of being "holy?"

because God is all holy & to be with Him is holy

Ephesians 1:4 also says that we were chosen to be "blameless." What does this week's memory verse say that Jesus did so that we could be blameless before God, even though we are prone to sin?

The resurrection of Jesus

How does 2 Corinthians 5:21 affirm this truth?

In 1 Corinthians 15:17, what does Paul tell us about the importance of the resurrection?

if Christ had not been raised we would still be in sin

In John 11:25, Jesus described Himself as the _resurrection_ and the _life_ . What other truth does Jesus affirm?

whoever believes in Jesus shall never die

How is that truth one of the "spiritual blessings" that Paul speaks about in Ephesians 1:3?

God has blessed us with every spiritual blessing in Christ

How is the fact that Jesus rose from the dead a reason for celebration every minute of every day?

because it gives us Grace & peace

How does Jesus' resurrection give you new birth and a living hope?

because through this we are given hope for our Tomorrows

> *Lord Jesus, You are the way, the truth and the life. If it were not for Your resurrection, I would have no hope for a better tomorrow and no cause for celebration. Thank You for paying the cost of my redemption! Amen.*

REFLECTION AND APPLICATION

Day 6

> *Lord Jesus, You call me to come away to a quiet place and rest. Help me honor Your request and spend time in Your presence each day. Amen.*

As part of this week's study, you examined a practice that Moses had, something the Bible calls "pitching a tent of meeting." On pages 22-24 of the *First Place 4 Health Member's Guide*, you are given some suggestions that will help you pitch your own tent of meeting—that place where you commune with God each day. Turn to that section of the *Member's Guide* and read those suggestions. On a separate piece of paper, make a sketch of your tent of meeting.

As you make this sketch, remember that considering the cost is part of the plans you make—so don't go beyond your budget limitations! Remember that it is the condition and desire of your heart, not the lavish surroundings, that are acceptable to God. What is important is that you are outside the mainstream of activity in your home and that the place you choose is comfortable and cozy. This is your place to meet with the Lord face to face, the way you would meet with a cherished friend.

As part of your sketch, make a list of the supplies that you will bring into your tent of meeting, and then make a list of all the other things that you will not allow inside your tent. (This could include things such as snacks and other foods that do not support your commitment to health and wellness, or even a radio or television or computer that will distract your attention.)

Share your tent sketch with your group during this week's meeting so that they can benefit from your ideas.

> *Thank You, Lord God, for energy, imagination and creativity. Thank You for inviting me to construct a tent of meeting where I can meet with You each day. Amen.*

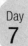

Day 7 REFLECTION AND APPLICATION

Lord God Almighty, I can only experience success because of Your great love for me. Thank You for Your mercy, compassion and grace. Amen.

This week's memory verse tells us that "in [God's] great mercy he has given us new birth and a living hope through the resurrection of Jesus Christ from the dead." Yet it is easy to say those words without giving any real thought to what they mean or how to apply them to our lives. In the space below, describe how each of the items listed applies to you and your success.

God's great mercy: _He is always ready with His_ _mercy if we ask & spend time with_ _Him._

New birth: _we are given new birth each_ _day through Her_

Living hope: _He not only gives us hope_ _but also grace for our praise_ _of Him_

The resurrection of Jesus Christ from the dead: _Jesus will come_ _back for us._

End your quiet time by thanking God for each of these things, which have been made possible because Jesus Christ was willing to pay the price of our redemption!

Thank You, Lord God, for bringing me into newness of life and for giving me the hope that because Jesus Christ rose from the dead, the same power that allowed Him to conquer sin and death now lives in me! Amen.

Group Prayer Requests

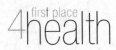

Today's Date: _4 - 24 - 14_

Name	Request
Tammy	for support through graduation
Shelly Long	treatment stage 3 cancer
Carol Hirsch	
Carol Sandbon	

Results

_____
_____
_____
_____
_____

celebrate our weakness

SCRIPTURE MEMORY VERSE
*But thanks be to God!
He gives us the victory through our Lord Jesus Christ.*
1 CORINTHIANS 15:57

The world would like you to believe that your greatest strength is having no weaknesses, no areas of personal vulnerability, and no flaws that leave you open to failure, ridicule or shame. However, Scripture presents a much different picture of those chosen by God to be His faithful servants. In contrast with the mentality of the world that a person's "greatest strength is having no weakness," read the words of the apostle Paul in 1 Corinthians 1:26-27. What does this passage tell you about your condition before the grace of God came into your life?

We were not wise or influential not noble birth

In 2 Corinthians 4:7, Paul gives another description of our human condition, even after the grace of God has appeared and saved us. What does this verse add to your understanding of 1 Corinthians 1:26-27?

sealed in jars of clay to show Gods power so that we can bring glory to Him

In what ways has God used your human weakness—the fact that you are a "jar of clay"—to show His all-surpassing power in and through you?

He uses me to tell others of His
great power & glory

As you begin this week's study, spend a few minutes thanking God that He has used your human weakness to show His all-surpassing power to those who still think strength is about having no areas of weakness.

Day 1 STRENGTH IN WEAKNESS

Gracious and loving Lord, I thank You that when I am weak, then I am strong, because You are my strength and my shield. Amen.

In 2 Corinthians 12:7-10, Paul describes a "weakness" (probably a physical malady) that afflicted him. Read that passage, and then in your own words summarize what Paul is telling us about this particular "thorn in the flesh."

We must always give God the glory
even in our weaknesses.

According to 2 Corinthians 12:7, why had Paul been given this affliction?

to keep him from becoming conceited

What does the word "torment" tell you about Paul's affliction?

Satan kept putting pressure on him

Whatever Paul's "thorn in the flesh" was, it was painful, powerful and persistent! Many of us also have a painful, powerful and persistent malady called compulsive overeating. In the space below, describe how this "thorn" is:

Painful: _We think we need something to eat to relive our hunger pains_

Powerful: _TV & others keep showing us all the things to eat_

Persistent: _our hunger pains don't go away_

Note that Paul says his thorn was "in the flesh." Do you think his pain was limited to the physical realm, or did it spill over into the other areas of his being? Explain your answer as you consider the connection between the physical, mental, emotional and spiritual aspects of life.

all of these are connected

How has compulsive overeating affected all four aspects of your being?

Physical: _I don't have the stamina to do things._

Mental: *I have to always be on guard against overeating*

Emotional: *I'm happier if I can lose the weight*

Spiritual: *I think I become stronger spiritually because I ask God to help me*

How is God's all-sufficient grace helping you experience victory?

when I ask He is there

Thank You, Lord, that in Your mercy and love You are helping me to put You first in all things in my life. I praise You for Your all-sufficient grace.

Day 2

WEAKNESS THAT LEADS TO STRENGTH

God, sometimes I get so overwhelmed by my troubles that I fail to see Your grace and mercy in and through the situation. Help me to see all the circumstances in my life from Your perspective. Amen.

Yesterday, we read about a "thorn in the flesh" that had been given to the apostle Paul. Recount what you learned about Paul's "thorn."

we can't expect our lives to always come easy. We must persist & allow God to do his work in us.

Second Corinthians 12:8 tells us that Paul asked _3_ times for the thorn to be removed. How did God answer Paul's prayer?

My grace is sufficient for you, for my power is made perfect in weakness

Second Corinthians 12:8 uses a specific word to describe Paul's prayer that the thorn be removed. What is that word, and what does the use of it tell you about the way Paul prayed?

pleaded – or begged

We also learn that God did not answer Paul's prayer in the way that Paul asked it to be answered. However, even though Paul did not receive the answer that *he* wanted in response to his plea, God did answer Paul! What does 2 Corinthians 12:9 tell us God said to Paul?

My grace is sufficient for you

How is the answer Paul received different from the worldview that tells us strength comes from having no weakness?

God's power is made perfect in weakness

What did Paul do in response to the answer he received from God?

He will boast more loudly

Second Corinthians 12:10 says that Paul had even learned to "delight" in his weakness. What truth allowed Paul to delight in his weakness?

For when I am weak then I am strong

How does Philippians 4:13 affirm the truth that Paul declares in 2 Corinthians 12:10?

I can do everything through Him who gives me the strength

What weakness do you have that is teaching you to rely more on God's strength? How can you rejoice in that weakness?

> *O Lord, You are my strength and my song. When I am weak, Your power can give me the strength I need to do the things You call me to do. Amen.*

Day 3 · UPSIDE DOWN

Great and merciful God, how thankful I am that You have chosen the weak in this world to be Your children, for if Your grace were dependent on my strength, I would be lost. Amen.

Somebody wisely said that a paradox is a truth standing on its head to get our attention. Throughout the pages of the Bible, we see God using paradox to teach us truths about the kingdom of God—a kingdom where things are topsy-turvy when compared to the beliefs and philosophies of the world.

John the Baptist, using the words of the prophet Isaiah to announce the coming of the long-awaited Messiah, told the Jewish people that Jesus was about to turn their world upside down. Turn in your Bible to Luke 3:4-6 and list all the things that were about to be turned upside down by the coming of the Lord.

every valley shall be filled
every mountain & hill made low
crooked roads become straight
the rough ways smooth
all mankind will see Gods salvation

Now turn to Luke 1:46-55. When Mary learned that she had been chosen to bring the Christ child into the world, she sang a beautiful song of thanksgiving and praise that we call "the Magnificat." In this song, she also sings about the things that will be turned upside down by this child she was carrying in her womb. Read Mary's song of praise, paying special attention to verses 51-53, and then list the reversals Mary talks about in her prophetic words.

God looks after the humble

Luke continues to show us this series of upside-down events about to take place when he tells us about the first sermon Jesus preached. Turn in your Bible to Luke 4:14-18 and read about what happened the day Jesus went into the synagogue on the Sabbath day. We are told that He began to speak by reading a passage from Isaiah's prophecy. In Luke 4:18, Jesus declares that the Spirit of the Lord is on Him and that because He is filled with the Spirit's power, He will do some very specific things for people the Jewish religious leaders considered lowly and undeserving of God's mercy and grace. Who are the four classes of people Jesus specifically names, and what does He say He will do for them?

Class of people	What Jesus says He will do for them
poor	preach good new
prisoners	proclaim freedom
blind	recovery of sight
oppressed	release them

In the introduction to this week's study, you looked at Paul's words in 1 Corinthians 1:26-27. Reread those verses. Even though Jesus had been crucified and had risen from the dead, He was and is still fulfilling the mission and purpose for which He was sent to earth. What kind of hope does that give you?

He is still doing His good work
_in me._

Gracious Lord, I am so thankful that You came to earth in human form to save those that society had cast aside as weak and useless. Because You are my Lord, I have hope, even in my weakness. Amen.

Day
4

DYING TO LIVE

Merciful Father, thank You for sending Jesus into the world to save me. How grateful I am that Your grace is not based on my strength but on Your strength being manifested in me. Amen.

Not only did Jesus' appearance turn the world upside down, but many of Jesus' teachings are also representative of the topsy-turvy world Jesus would usher in with His coming. Listed on the chart below are some of the paradoxical statements we find in the Gospels and Epistles. Complete the "I must" section of each line.

Scripture	If I want to . . .	I must . . .
Luke 9:24-26	save my life	first lose it
Luke 22:26-27	rule	rule like the one who serves
John 12:24	produce fruit	die to produce good
Rom. 8:13	live	put to death the misdeeds
2 Cor. 12:9-10	be strong	delight in weakness
Jas. 4:10	be lifted up	humble ourselves

As you look over your list, identify two things you want in your life today. Circle both of these, along with the "I must . . ." that accompanies the corresponding "If I want to. . ." List the two "wants" below, and then write about what you must do in order to have those things in your life. Note that these truths apply to the spiritual plane of your life in Christ, not the physical realm, so put each statement into the proper perspective as you describe both the "want" and the "must do." For example, if you want to increase the kingdom of God by making disciples, you must die to your self-wants and be willing to be used by God (see John 12:24).

1. _____

_____

2. _____

_____

Merciful God, thank You for giving me Your Word and Your truth. Help
me to be a diligent worker who searches Your truth in order to discover all
the wisdom Your words contain. Amen.

A PARADOXICAL VICTORY

Lord, thank You for choosing me to be a vessel of Your truth and love.
Thank You for all the spiritual blessings You have given me in Christ Jesus.

This week, we have examined the concept of paradox—truth standing on
its head to get our attention. Summarize what you have learned about
paradox and why spiritual truths about the kingdom of God were presented in paradoxical fashion.

_____

_____

_____

_____

This week's memory verse is also a paradoxical statement. However, in
order to understand the topsy-turvy nature of the apostle Paul's words,
we have to look at this verse in the context of the larger passage in which
it is found. Turn in your Bible and read 1 Corinthians 15:50-57. What is
the paradox being presented in Paul's words?

_____

_____

_____

_____

In 1 Corinthians 15:51, Paul says that he is telling his readers a mystery.
Based on what you have learned this week, how does the Bible use paradox to tell you about the mystery of God's grace?

The perishable can not enherit the
kingdom of God

Up to the time when Jesus came into the world to turn the religious establishment upside down, the people were bound by the covenant of the law. What does 1 Corinthians 15:56 tell you about the law?

the power of sin is the law

What happens when we try to "earn" our salvation by perfectly keeping the law rather than humbly accepting God's grace and acknowledging that we are flawed human beings?

give yourself fully to the work of the Lord

Paul makes a bold statement in 1 Corinthians 15:54: "Death has been swallowed up in victory." If trying to perfectly keep the law results in death, where does our victory come from?

from the Lord

After making the bold affirmation that our victory comes through our Lord Jesus Christ, Paul goes on to say what our response to this marvelous grace needs to be. Read 1 Corinthians 15:58 and summarize what Paul is saying in this verse.

Stand firm always give yourself fully to the Work of the Lord

End your quiet time by writing your own Magnificat—your own song of praise—for the wonderful things that God has done for you in Christ Jesus. (If you are musically inclined, you might want to sing rather than write your words on paper!)

God
You alway seem to come to me with your works even if they are not what I have ask for. Your know what I need even before I ask.

O Lord God, today I sing Your praise, for You have done great things for me. Your name is holy and Your love is beyond measure. Thank You for choosing me to be a vessel of Your truth and grace. Amen.

Day 6 | REFLECTION AND APPLICATION

Thank You, loving Lord, for Your Word and Your promises. Thank You that in Christ Jesus, all the words You have spoken are "yes" and "amen."

During the Day Three study this week, you looked at four classes of people to whom Jesus came to minister: the poor, prisoners, the blind and the oppressed. As you look at each of these classes of people, it is important to put them in proper perspective. In Luke's Gospel:

- **The poor** are the marginalized—those excluded from social and religious interaction because of gender, age, economic position, physical malady or religious impurity.

- **The prisoners** who will be released are those who need to be freed from the personal problems that keep them living in darkness and despair and that keep them from being faithful and fruitful servants.

- **The blind** are those who have not seen the truth of the gospel of Jesus Christ.

- **The oppressed** are those who have given in to temptation and have consequently become bound to destructive ways of living.

Select one of the four categories above that might describe your situation at the present time. (All four may apply, or none may apply.) Consider how Jesus Christ came to turn your situation upside down. This week's memory verse affirms that He came to give you victory. Using the pages of your prayer journal, spend time talking to God about how Jesus has the power to take any weakness and turn it into strength.

Gracious God, I often feel oppressed. I have given in to temptation too many times and, as a result, I have become bound by destructive habit patterns. Thank You for helping me realize the truth that victory is mine in Christ Jesus my Lord. Amen.

REFLECTION AND APPLICATION

Day 7

Lord God, You made me for Yourself. Help me to honor You with my body, even as I rejoice in Your goodness and tender mercy. Amen.

This week's memory verse talks about victory, but as we have seen this week, this is not a victory that we can claim in our own strength and power. Jesus Christ is the victorious one! In His goodness and tender mercy, He allows those who believe in His name to celebrate His victory over sin and death along with Him. As you consider what it is to celebrate success, who is it that really deserves the honor and glory for all your daily victories and small successes?

To worship is to give God the glory and honor due Him. We are called to worship God with our bodies by caring for them in a way that honors the Creator of all things. On this day of reflection, worship God by exercising the wonderfully made body God fashioned just for you. As you exercise and get increasingly more fit, remember that your true strength is not about physical prowess but about relying on God's strength to shore up your weakness. Make your exercise time today a time of joyful celebration as you meditate on the victory that is yours in Christ Jesus your Lord.

Thank You, thank You! O Lord, You have been so good to me. You have given me a physical body, and You have filled me with joy and hope. Today I will celebrate Your goodness and grace. Amen.

Group Prayer Requests

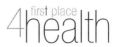

Today's Date: _5 - 1 - 14_

Name	Request
Harchant	
Eugene Mann	
Missionaries	

Results

_____

_____

_____

_____

_____

_____

Week Five

celebrate
unity

In Ephesians 4:2-6, the apostle Paul declared, "Be completely humble and gentle; be patient, bearing with one another in love. Make every effort to keep the unity of the Spirit through the bond of peace. There is one body and one Spirit—just as you were called to one hope when you were called—one Lord, one faith . . . one God and Father of all, who is over all and through all and in all." With those words, Paul began to teach the first-generation Christians in Ephesus what it really meant to live in unity with their brothers and sisters in Christ.

Notice that Paul did not use the word "cooperation," nor did he talk about negotiation or "agreeing to disagree." Paul used the word "unity," and he did so for a very specific reason. As believers, we are one Body— the Body of the Lord Jesus Christ. Christ Himself is the head of the Body. We share one Spirit and have one common goal: the goal of doing God's work here on earth.

As you begin this week's study, you will focus on the value and benefits of being connected to a group of people who hold the same values and beliefs as you do. This is extremely important as you make progress on your wellness journey, as surrounding yourself with a support system is a critical component that helps you acheive success in your goals.

UNIFIED EFFORT

*Lord God, open my eyes to those around me and show me the
value of those individuals You have placed in my life. Amen.*

Look at Mark 2:1-5. In this story, Jesus has returned to the town of Capernaum. What kind of reception did He receive?

Many gathered

Why do you think the people were so anxious to see Him?

*They heard he had come home &
was going to preach the word to them*

Look closer at verses 3 and 4. What motivated the four friends as they carried their friend to Jesus?

their friends condition was desperate

The four men were certainly united in the goal, and their working together resulted in a good and pleasant outcome for their friend. Have you considered the role you play as you relate to others around you?

Would you be willing to go to that much effort to introduce someone to Jesus? Why or why not?

_____

_____

_____

_____

As you saw in the introduction to this week's study, Paul begins teaching on unity in the Body with some instructions on how believers are to act toward others in the Body. Read Ephesians 4:1 and see what Paul is urging his readers to do:

We are to live a life _worthy_ of the _calling_ we have _received_.

Turn to 1 John 3:18 and read the instructions given there to believers. How are we to love others?

with actions & truth

_____

_____

_____

Is there a "unified action" you need to take toward someone in your circle of friends that will move her or him toward an encounter with Jesus? If so, what is that action?

_____

_____

_____

_____

*Gracious and loving Lord, help me love others in truth
and action and not just in words. Amen.*

UNITY BRINGS HOPE

Lord, at times this thing called unity is hard to achieve. Help me understand how I can live in harmony with my brothers and sisters in Christ. Amen.

Read Mark 2:1-5 again and try to envision what was happening in Capernaum. Jesus was teaching the Word (see v. 2), and so many people had gathered to see and hear Him that there was no room in the house to hold everyone. Yet despite the crowds, these four friends were determined to bring their sick friend to Jesus.

We can only imagine what Jesus thought as He saw four men lowering their friend on a stretcher through the roof. He may have been in the middle of teaching, when all of a sudden He began to hear a commotion on the roof and then witnessed a most unusual chain of events. The owner of the house was probably dismayed and in a state of shock. But more than likely, it brought Jesus great pleasure to see such a bold move of friendship and unity among those friends.

What was it about these four men that prompted Jesus to heal their paralytic friend (see v. 5)?

their faith

Notice that not only was the sick man healed physically, but he was also healed spiritually—his sins were forgiven. If you read on in Mark 2:11-13, you will see that the unity and faith of these friends also brought hope to the crowds that witnessed such a miracle. Describe a time when you were blessed to witness friendship in action that not only brought hope to yourself but to others.

Can you think of a current situation in your life that is in need of such faith in the healing power of Jesus?

_____

_____

_____

_____

> *Lord God, how thankful I am that You are loving and forgiving and patient with me, even when I am not patient with myself. Thank You for giving me this new day, created for my enjoyment. Amen.*

Day 3 · UNITY BRINGS COMFORT

Sovereign Lord, today I am becoming more mindful of the struggle that goes on inside of me and others. Help me find a way to be a comfort to others as You have comforted me. Amen.

Neosporin is an antibacterial ointment that kills germs and at the same times makes a wound feel better. That's what we need to be in the Body of Christ. Can you imagine treating a wound with alcohol instead of peroxide?! We don't want to inflict pain on each other.

Read 2 Corinthians 1:2-8. How is God described in these verses?

Father of compassion
God of comfort

_____

_____

What should be your motivation as you seek to be a source of comfort to others?

faith in God

_____

_____

As we work with others in community, we can be a unified source of comfort to those around us. Whether it is to meet a financial, physical or spiritual need, God can use us to be a comfort to others. Describe a person you know who is going through a difficult time. What could you do to offer comfort to that person today?

_____

_____

_____

_____

_____

Something amazing happens when we decide to be a comfort to others. Read Isaiah 58:6-12. In this passage, the people of Israel were hurting and were trying to get God to notice them by engaging in a meaningless fast. Their hearts were not in it, and they were quarreling amongst themselves. They were not sincere in their fast. The Lord was calling for a different kind of fast. What does He tell them to do in verses 6-7?

1. _loose_ the chains of injustice

2. set the oppressed _free_ and break every _yoke_

3. share your _food_ with the hungry and provide the poor wanderer with _shelter_

4. _clothe_ the naked and do not turn away from your own _flesh_ and _blood_.

In verses 8-12, the Lord gives a long list of what they can expect from Him if they are obedient and do these things. List some of these below.

You will have light

healing will appear

be righteousness

God glory will guard you

call & the Lord will answer

This was certainly not the kind of fast the people had in mind. God wanted them to fast from their abundance and minister to the needs of others out of their overflow. In looking back at this day's lesson, is God directing you to minister to someone in a particular way? Identify that person and the way He wants you to be a source of comfort to him or her.

_____

_____

_____

_____

Spend the remainder of your quiet time praising God for the great comfort He has given to you. Thank God for the Spirit that allows you to be a source of comfort to others.

> *I love you, O Lord, my strength! Without You, I would be mired in self-obsessed behavior. Through Your Spirit, I can be kind, loving and generous toward others. Thank You for Your good gifts to me. Amen.*

Day 4 — UNITY BRINGS MATURITY

O Lord, I know that You desire that I grow in grace and knowledge.
Help me to be humble and submissive as I listen to Your Word
so that I can grow up in my faith. Amen.

At the end of the passage on unity we studied earlier this week, Paul said that the goal is our unity—whether that unity is within ourselves or with our brothers and sisters in Christ. Read Ephesians 4:11-13 and summarize what Paul says in this passage as it applies to unity and maturity.

we all have different needs & God will show us the way for our own particular needs.

Paul is describing how God gave the people of His Church spiritual gifts (such as apostles, prophets, evangelists, teachers and pastors) for the purpose of preparing the Body of Christ for works of service and encouraging one another, so that they may be unified and mature in their knowledge of Christ Jesus. Continue reading Ephesians 4:14-16. What results from this gifting of the Church (see v. 14)?

we will no longer be infants in our faith we will grow into him

Because of the dedicated teaching and shepherding of leaders in the Church, we are unified as a Body and can grow to be mature in our knowledge of the teachings of Christ. In Ephesians 4:15, Paul provides the imagery that all believers "grow up into him who is the Head, that is, Christ." What does verse 16 tell you about your role in the Body of Christ, His Church?

we grow & build itself up in love as each part does work

We all have specific roles to play. Just as God has gifted the Church with pastors and teachers, He has gifted each of us with spiritual gifts as well. These could include the gifts already mentioned, but they could also include the gifts of mercy, hospitality, leadership or administration (just to name a few). What role(s) do you feel that you play at this time within the Body of Christ? Are your God-given gifts being used and bearing fruit for His kingdom?

The most obvious characteristic about the Body of Christ is that we need one another. Together, working as one, we can support each other in love and truly grow up in our faith so that we become more like Jesus—the Head of our Body!

Gracious God, thank You for Your Word and Your truth. Thank You that I can practice my faith so that I can become mature in Christ and be able to serve You to the best of my God-given ability. Amen.

Day 5

A RECIPE FOR UNITY

My Lord and my God, it is my desire to please You. Yet I can only bring my actions in sync with my desires through Your might and power. O Lord God, please help me. Amen.

As we saw in yesterday's lesson, we can be a part of bringing goodness to the lives of those around us. One important element to being motivated is that we must experience unity within ourselves. When we are fragmented (which is the opposite of united) within our own being, either one part rules or all parts fail. Unity is elusive.

Think about the parts of your own being. Does one part rule? Or do all parts fail? Listed below are the aspects of the four-sided person. As you look at these four aspects of your being, decide whether: (1) that quadrant rules the other three; or (2) that quadrant is being oppressed by one of the other parts.

Body	Mind
Emotions	Spirit

Write your findings beside each aspect of your being that you listed. In light of what you have just discovered, reread Ephesians 4:2. In this verse, Paul lists four specific things that can help you achieve unity, whether it is inner unity or unity with the other members of the Body of Christ. List those four specific things Paul says you need to be to achieve unity.

1. _be humble_
2. _" gentle_
3. _" patient_
4. _" bearing with one another_

Ephesians 4:3 tells you how to use these four things. What do the words "make every effort" mean to you?

push hard work together

Now look back at the list of four things we are called to be in order to achieve "unity." How can those four ways of being help you achieve unity within yourself? In other words, how can you be completely humble, gentle, and patient, bearing with yourself in love? (This question is key to your success in ministering to others, so please give it careful thought!)

How can your body be completely humble, gentle and patient, bearing with your mind, emotions and spirit in love?

give our whole being to God

How can your mind be completely humble, gentle and patient, bearing with your body, emotions and spirit in love?

always think before we act

How can your emotions be completely humble, gentle and patient, bearing with your body, mind and spirit in love?

Think positive & be happy

How can your spirit be completely humble, gentle and patient, bearing with your body, mind and emotions in love?

> *Lord God, help me to be completely humble, gentle and patient,*
> *bearing with all the various parts of this body You created. Amen.*

Day
6

REFLECTION AND APPLICATION

Sovereign and merciful God, in love and mercy, You set me free.
Even though I am still beset by internal conflicts, I will be of good cheer,
for You have overcome the world. Amen.

Yesterday, you looked at how to begin to bring all parts of your personality and your own being into unity. As you have probably discovered, inner unity is not an easy undertaking! However, achieving inner unity is essential to your success in any endeavor—especially in your journey to lead a healthier life. As you reflect on what you have learned thus far this week, what is the greatest challenge you face in achieving unity?

> *to have my mind go along with my body with my eating & exercise*

Throughout his writings, the apostle Paul used the little word "therefore" to describe an amazing truth that comes from the teaching he has just given. Romans 8:1 contains one of those "therefore" moments. After expounding on the internal struggle between what we want to do and what we actually do in Romans 7:14-24, Paul gives us the solution to our dilemma in Romans 7:25. Reread that verse and express in your own words what Paul is saying.

> *Through Jesus Christ the Lord we can achieve complete unity*

Then in Romans 8:1, we see the word "therefore" followed by a truth so profound that it is almost beyond our ability to comprehend. Write the truth of Romans 8:1 in the space below:

> *if we are in Jesus Christ there is no condemnation*

Spend the rest of your reflection time today allowing this truth to sink into the depths of your soul. Yes, the internal conflicts still rage. Yes, you still do things you don't want to do. But thanks be to God! For those who are in Christ Jesus, there is no condemnation! End your meditation time by asking yourself the question: What impact does this truth—the fact that there is no condemnation—have on me?

Lord Jesus, You died for me. You took the punishment. I get the privilege of being a beloved child of God. Thank You for coming to my rescue. Amen.

Day 7 REFLECTION AND APPLICATION

How blessed I am that You are my God! How thankful I am for Your goodness to me. When I was still a sinner, Christ died for me! Amen.

This week, we have looked at the importance of having a unified group of people to support us and understanding the comfort we are created to give others in Christ Jesus. We have also examined the importance of Christian maturity as the path to unity, both within ourselves and in relation to others in the Body of Christ. Review your work from day to day and pick one Christian value that you need to "put on" in greater measure to help you dwell with others in unity. What behavior will you need to let go of in order to grasp this new way of responding to the needs of others?

be patient

give others encouragement

After you have identified the good and pleasing way you can dwell with others in unity, collect a collage of pictures from magazines, or any other source, that depict this way of living. Paste these illustrations on a piece of heavy-weight paper and hang your picture by your front door so that you will remember to be as healing to others as a comforting ointment when you go out into the world as an ambassador of Jesus Christ.

Merciful Father, You call me to be an ambassador of Christ. Help me to always adorn myself with behavior fitting one called to carry the message of God's grace. Amen.

Group Prayer Requests

first place
4health

Today's Date: _____

Name	Request

Results

_____
_____
_____
_____
_____
_____

celebrate patience and preparation

SCRIPTURE MEMORY VERSE
*I say to myself, "The LORD is my portion;
therefore I will wait for him."*
LAMENTATIONS 3:24

One of the central themes that run throughout the pages of the Bible is patience—God's patience with us and our need to be patient with the process as God does His good work in and through us.

Often, instead of valuing the Christian virtue of patience, we strain at the bit. We choose not to walk in sync with the Spirit and, consequently, we fail to enjoy the wonderful rhythm of God's grace. "Wait for the Lord" is a command—not an option—for those who have chosen to follow the Lord!

As you begin this week's study, turn in your Bible to Psalm 40:1 and read David's words, paying close attention to the sequence of events:

I waited patiently for the LORD;
he turned to me and heard my cry.

Note the passion in the last word in the verse: *cry*. David was crying out to the Lord! This was not an idle request; it was a passionate plea. Yet even in his state of mind, David waited patiently on the Lord. David's stance differs radically from the instant gratification mentality that characterizes the world in which we live.

PATIENT IN AFFLICTION

Day 1

O Lord, You are my help and my deliverer! In You I put my trust.
Please hear my voice and come to my assistance. Amen.

Turn again to Psalm 40:1 and notice that sequence of events that led to David's deliverance. Write out that sequence below:

_____ waited _____ for the _____.

The _____ turned _____ David.

The _____ heard _____ _____.

In Psalm 34:15, what did the Lord turn toward David? (Two things are listed in this verse, so list the choice that has to do with hearing.)

_____

_____

_____

Psalm 34:17 tells us what happens when the righteous cry out to the Lord. Again, there are two things listed in this verse. This time, write them both down.

_____

_____

_____

_____

Now turn your attention to Psalm 34:18. Where is the Lord when you are brokenhearted?

_____

_____

_____

_____

Still focusing on Psalm 34:18, what does the Lord do for those who are crushed in spirit?

_____

_____

_____

_____

What is the promise given in Psalm 34:22?

_____

_____

_____

_____

What does Psalm 34:19 tell you about "the righteous" and "trouble"?

_____

_____

_____

_____

Psalm 34:19-20 is not only a precious truth for those who cry out to the Lord today, but it was also a prophecy of what would happen to Jesus, God's Son. Turn in your Bible to John 19:28-37 to see how this prophecy was fulfilled. What did you discover?

_____

_____

_____

_____

What does John 19:28-37 tell you about God's ability to use human circumstances to bring His Word to pass?

_____

_____

_____

What does confidence in God's Word and in His promises have to do with patience?

_____

_____

_____

_____

_____

Lord God, today I will meditate on Your Word, confident that everything You have promised will come to pass in Your perfect time and way. Amen.

CRYING OUT TO GOD

Day 2

Sovereign Lord, so often I grow impatient with Your timing. Help me to take delays as opportunities to learn more about You. Amen.

Prayer sets spiritual forces in motion, although the immediate effect is often invisible, perhaps for a long time. In Daniel 9:1-4, the prophet Daniel is in exile and is looking to God's Word for relief. Read Daniel 9:1-4, and then describe the circumstance that led to Daniel's prayer.

_____

_____

_____

_____

_____

Had Daniel not believed in the trustworthiness and truth of God's Word, would he have had any hope for the restoration of Jerusalem? How is what you read in Daniel 9:1-4 like what we read in Psalm 34:19-20?

_____

_____

_____

_____

Daniel 9:3 tells us that Daniel, like David, "turned to the Lord God and pleaded with him in prayer and petition." And as Daniel prayed, he did something else. What does Daniel 9:4 tell you that he did?

_____

_____

_____

Read Daniel's beautiful prayer of confession as listed in Daniel 9:4-19. How is the prayer that Daniel prayed similar or different to the prayers you normally pray?

_____

_____

_____

_____

Notice that Daniel does not begin his prayer with a request or confession of his sins. Read Daniel 9:4. How did Daniel begin his prayer?

_____

_____

_____

After praising God, what does Daniel do next (see vv. 5-6)?

_____

_____

_____

Does Daniel blame God for the fate of the Israelites, who are now in exile? (You will find the answer in Daniel 9:9-14.) What does Daniel say about God in verse 9?

_____

_____

_____

_____

What does Daniel appeal to in verses 16-17?

_____

_____

_____

Daniel ends his prayer by asking God to hear him, to forgive and to act. On what basis does Daniel make this appeal, according to verse 18?

_____

_____

_____

_____

Pick one element of Daniel's confessional prayer that you would like to incorporate into your own prayer life. Then, in the pages of your journal, offer up that prayer to God using Daniel's prayer as a template.

Gracious and merciful God, I do not make requests of You because I am righteous, but because You are merciful and loving. Thank You for forgiving my sins. Amen.

AN ANSWER HAS BEEN GIVEN

Day 3

Lord, You are righteous in all Your ways and loving in all You do. Even though I get impatient with You, You never give up on me. Thank You for Your tender mercies. Amen.

Yesterday, you looked at Daniel's heartfelt prayer of confession. What portion of Daniel's prayer did the Holy Spirit especially illuminate for you, and why do you think that was so?

_____

_____

_____

_____

Daniel's prayer was sincere and heartfelt. It contained all the elements of prayer that make our prayers acceptable to God. Name three of the aspects of Daniel's prayer that you remember from yesterday:

1. _____

2. _____

3. _____

Daniel 9:20-23 tells us that God heard Daniel's prayer. Read those verses now and describe what happened as Daniel was praying.

_____
_____
_____
_____

Now look at Daniel 10:12. When were spiritual forces set in motion to bring Daniel's requests to fruition?

_____
_____
_____
_____

Scripture says that from the first day Daniel began to pray, his words were heard. Yet the answer to Daniel's prayer did not materialize for 70 years! Gabriel told Daniel that the answer he was seeking was a work in progress. And although that progress began the moment Daniel began to pray—even though the spiritual forces had been set in motion—it took a very long time before the results were visible on a human level. Times of mourning, solitude, weakness and fear were required before the answer eventually came to pass. Yet Daniel remained steadfastly confident that his prayers had been heard and God was orchestrating all things together to grant Daniel's request.

How does the story of Daniel help you understand the meaning of the words "patient endurance"?

_____
_____
_____
_____
_____

What does Daniel's story tell you about remaining steadfastly confident, even though your First Place 4 Health results may not be visible on a human level for some months?

_____
_____
_____
_____
_____

How does this truth help you understand why it is important to commit a year to the process?

_____
_____
_____
_____
_____

A wonderful promise to claim during the waiting period is found in Philippians 1:6. Read that verse now, and claim the promise that God will complete the good work He has begun in you. You might want to write this verse on an index card and carry it with you as a reminder that spiritual forces have been set in motion that will ensure your success!

> God, how precious are Your thoughts of me. Your plans for me are good.
> You know the end from the beginning. Today, I will put my trust in You.

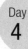

Day
4

THE IMPORTANCE OF PREPARATION

Gracious God, I know You are in control of all things at all times.
I pray that my mind and heart will be in agreement so that I can be
assured of Your love and grace. Amen.

For the past two days, we have been studying Daniel, a Jewish exile who was living in Babylon. Even though Daniel was far away from Jerusalem, he never lost faith in the God of Israel. He waited patiently as God put spiritual forces in motion that would eventually bring the answer to his prayers. God used another Jewish exile, a beautiful Jewish girl living in Susa, the capital of Persia, to bring deliverance to His people living in that foreign land. As you can probably guess, that young Jewish girl's name was Esther. Through a set of circumstances that only God could have orchestrated, Esther was in the right place at the right time—and willing to do what was required of her.

In Esther 4:14, we are told what Esther's cousin, Mordecai, said to his adopted daughter, who in God's providence had become the queen of Persia. The Jews were facing annihilation when he asked Esther to use her influence with the king to save her people. Exactly what did Mordecai say to Esther?

_____

_____

_____

Esther had come to this position for such a time as this! Yet prior to being used by God in this powerful way, Esther had gone through a season of preparation. Read about the beauty regimen Esther went through before being brought before the king in Esther 2:12. How long was Esther's season of preparation?

_____

_____

_____

Another example of preparation prior to service is found in the story of the apostle Paul. We know that Paul experienced a dramatic conversion on the Damascus road, but he did not immediately go into ministry. Read Galatians 1:11-24, and then describe the preparation Paul went through before beginning his ministry to the Gentiles.

_____

_____

_____

_____

Galatians 1:15 tells us that God had set Paul apart from _____. But Paul was not called into God's service until God's time was right— and until he had gone through the necessary preparation. How long was it before Paul went to Jerusalem to get acquainted with Peter and the other disciples (see v. 18)?

_____

_____

_____

Perhaps God is preparing you for an exciting new area of ministry. What might God be preparing you to do? (Read 2 Corinthians 1:3-4 for some ideas about how God is planning to use you!)

_____

_____

_____

_____

According to this passage, why does God comfort us in our affliction?

_____

_____

_____

_____

In an earlier week of study, we looked at how God uses our weakness so that His strength might be displayed in us. How does 2 Corinthians 1:3-4 affirm that truth?

_____

_____

_____

Thank You, merciful God, for comforting me and then calling me to comfort others with the comfort I have received from You. Amen.

Day 5 — MY PORTION

Gracious God, You are my portion, and I will wait for You in confidence that at the proper time You will answer my heartfelt prayers. Amen.

The memory verse for this week gives us yet another reason for waiting for God's will and way. Write this week's memory verse below.

_____

_____

_____

Why is Jeremiah, the writer of Lamentations, willing to wait for the Lord?

_____

_____

_____

In order to fully understand what is being said in your memory verse, you must put it into the context in which it appears in the Bible. Turn to Lamentations 3 and read verses 19-26. What was going on in Jeremiah's life when these verses were written? Was this a pleasant time for Jeremiah? Give specifics to support your answer.

_____

_____

_____

According to Lamentations 3:21-23, where does Jeremiah say that his hope comes from?

_____

_____

_____

_____

How does Psalm 121:1-2 affirm this truth?

_____

_____

_____

_____

Continue reading in Psalm 121. What do verses 3-6 tell us that the Lord does for us?

_____

_____

_____

_____

Yes, the Lord watches over us. He is our shade in the daytime and our guardian at night! Psalm 121:8 even tells us *when* the Lord watches over us. What are those times?

_____

_____

_____

Now turn to Psalm 73:25-26. How do these verses agree with what is being said in this week's memory verse?

_____

_____

_____

_____

Psalm 119:57 adds another dimension to the truth found in this week's memory verse. What is the desired outcome when the Lord is our portion?

_____

_____

_____

_____

How is studying God's Word and seeking to live a healthy life part of the obedience that says the Lord is our portion forever?

_____

_____

_____

_____

O Lord, You are my portion, and I seek You with all my heart.
My heart is content when I find my rest in You. Amen.

Day 6

REFLECTION AND APPLICATION

The earth is filled with Your love, O Lord. How thankful I am that You chose me before the foundation of the earth and You are preparing me for the good work You have created me to achieve. Amen.

This week, we looked at the prayer Daniel prayed on behalf of God's people when they were in exile and examined the various elements of that prayer. In your *First Place 4 Health Member's Guide*, you are given the acrostic F.I.R.S.T. as a template for your prayers. Reread Daniel 9:4-19, and then turn to pages 26-27 in the *Member's Guide* to read the explanation of the F.I.R.S.T. acrostic. Next, write the verse numbers in Daniel's prayer that correspond with each letter in the acrostic F.I.R.S.T.

Focus: _____

Invite: _____

Reconcile: _____

Surrender: _____

Trust: _____

(Note that there are at least two verses for each word, and you will be able to find more if you do a thorough search.)

> *Gracious God, today I will trust in You and Your Word. I know that even though it may take time, patience and preparation, You are working all things together for Your glory and my good. Amen.*

REFLECTION AND APPLICATION

Day 7

Thank You, Lord God, for comforting me when I am afflicted and then calling me to extend that same comfort to others in their time of need.

We often wonder what God is calling us to do in His kingdom. Sometimes, we may even doubt that God has a plan and purpose for our life. Yet Scripture presents an encouraging picture of the usefulness of those who have been saved by God's grace. We are all called to be ambassadors of God and tell the world that God is no longer counting our sins against us (see 2 Corinthians 5:20)!

On this day of reflection, review the lessons you have learned this week as you sit quietly before God, asking Him what He is preparing you to do. Jeremiah 29:11 gives you great assurance about God's plans. As you reflect on those words, ask God to begin to reveal to you what He has in store for you, knowing that He is your portion and His plan for you is good.

Be sure to factor in the comfort you have received from God, because Scripture tells us that God asks us to comfort others in the same ways that He has comforted us. Close your meditation time with a psalm or song of praise. (Psalm 100 is a wonderful psalm to read, but if you are musically inclined, you can sing a praise song instead.)

What comfort have you received recently from God?

_____

_____

_____

Based on what you have learned this week, what might God's good plan for you be?

_____

_____

_____

_____

What preparation will you need to go through before God can use you as His ambassador, or continue to use you in even more powerful ways?

_____

_____

_____

_____

Gracious and loving God, Your compassions are new every morning and Your faithfulness is great. You are my portion, and I will wait patiently for You. Amen.

Group Prayer Requests

first place
4health

Today's Date: _____

Name	Request

Results

_____
_____
_____
_____
_____
_____

celebrate God's dwelling place

SCRIPTURE MEMORY VERSE
Do not defile the land where you live and where I dwell,
for I, the LORD, dwell among the Israelites.
NUMBERS 35:34

"Since we have these promises, dear friends, let us purify ourselves from everything that contaminates body and spirit, perfecting holiness out of reverence for God," declared the apostle Paul in 2 Corinthians 7:1. The apostle Peter echoed these thoughts: "Dear friends, I urge you, as aliens and strangers in the world, to abstain from sinful desires, which war against your soul" (1 Peter 2:11). A theme that runs throughout the pages of the Bible, repeated in many different ways, is the admonition to take good care of the things that are precious to God.

How do both Paul and Peter address their readers in the verses cited?

_____

_____

_____

What does the phrase "dear friends" tell you about the sincerity of Paul and Peter in writing these words?

_____

_____

_____

Have you ever considered yourself a dear friend of the saints that have gone before you—those who have traveled the path, learned from their mistakes and taken the time to write down the lessons they have learned from God, for your benefit? Why or why not?

_____

_____

_____

_____

_____

Perhaps nowhere is the consequences of caring for God's Temple, the place where God dwells, more vividly illustrated than in the little book of Haggai. Although 18 years had passed since the exiled Jews had been allowed to return to Jerusalem, God's house still remained in ruins. It seems that the people were so busy doing their own thing that they did not have enough time to care for the one thing that was important to God. And God was not pleased! Through the prophet Haggai, God invited the people to "give careful thought to [their] ways" (Haggai 1:7). This week, we will accept the challenge from our dear friend Haggai and "give careful thought to our ways" when it comes to caring for the place where God dwells.

THE PROBLEM WITH PROCRASTINATION

Day 1

Lord God, it is so easy to put off until tomorrow what I know I should do today. Forgive me for those times when I know what to do but don't do it.

"Procrastination" is a word with which most of us are all too familiar. Putting off until tomorrow what we know we need to do today is a universal problem that existed long before God sent Haggai to give the Jews a wake-up call! The problem with procrastination is that when we put off those things that we know God wants us to do, we are not making His priorities our priorities.

God sent the Old Testament prophets to comfort the afflicted and afflict the comfortable. Read the words of the prophet Haggai in Haggai 1:1-5. What type of message did God give to the prophet to give to His people?

_____

_____

_____

_____

_____

Now read Haggai 1:2. What were the people saying that displeased God?

_____

_____

_____

Were God's people neglecting the rebuilding of God's house out of ignorance? Explain your answer.

_____

_____

_____

_____

In ancient Israel, the Temple was where God dwelt among His people. Consequently, the condition of the Temple was a reflection of the honor and respect the people had toward God. It was a clear indicator of their relationship with Him. Haggai tells us that the Israelites lived in the shadow of the Temple ruins as they scurried about their own affairs. Who were the Israelites putting first when they focused on their own wants and desires while neglecting God's house?

_____

_____

_____

_____

Are you neglecting something that God wants you to do? If God were to send Haggai to you, what would he say about the things you may be doing that are keeping you from fully honoring God by caring for the body in which His Holy Spirit makes His home? Write what He might say to you below.

_____ [your name], you are saying the time has not yet come for

_____

_____ .

Father, You invite me to consider my ways and bring my priorities in line with Yours. Help me to honor You by caring for the things that are important to You.

GIVE CAREFUL THOUGHT TO YOUR WAYS

Day **2**

O Lord God Almighty, You invite me to give careful thought to my ways so that Your words and my actions are in sync. Help me show my love for You by being obedient to Your revealed will. Amen.

Haggai came with a specific message for God's people. Turn to Haggai 1:5 and write God's plea below:

Give _____ _____ to your _____ .

What is significant about the fact that God repeats those same words in verse 7?

_____

_____

_____

All believers have the Holy Spirit dwelling within them to guide them into all truth. Everything we need to know to live a life pleasing to God has been revealed to us in the pages of God's written Word. Through the power of the Holy Spirit, God brings those words into our awareness in a variety of ways. Listed in the chart that follows are the five primary ways in which God speaks to His people today. Next to each of the ways God speaks, list the ways that you are hearing His voice.

God speaks to me through . . .	How God is using this to speak to me
His written Word	
My prayer time	
The words of believers	
My life circumstances	
My heartfelt desires and visions	

Often we say that we want to hear God's voice, but we need to consider if we have taken action on the things that God has already revealed to us. It is not that we do not hear God; sometimes we hear Him, but we neglect to do the things He tells us are important to Him. We need to remember that one small act of obedience is more pleasing to God than all of our great intentions. List one thing you can do today to bring your life in sync with God's Word.

_____

_____

_____

_____

Psalm 95:7-8 reminds us that if we hear God's voice today, we are not to harden our hearts. There is no valid reason to put off until tomorrow what you have been called to do today. Write a prayer committing the action you believe God is telling you to do today, and then do your part by following through with that commitment.

_____

_____

_____

_____

_____

Gracious and loving Lord, I hear You saying, "The time has come."
What You want me to do is clear. By the power of the Holy Spirit, help
me to take one small, obedient step this day. Amen.

WHEN THERE IS NEVER ENOUGH | Day 3

Lord, I know that I should not neglect the things that are important
to You, and I want to please You with all my heart. Help me to
respond to Your words in joyful obedience. Amen.

In response to the procrastination expressed by the people, God instructed Haggai to ask them a question designed to express His frustration with their lack of action. Read Haggai 1:3-4, and then describe the nature of God's complaint.

_____

_____

_____

_____

It was not a matter of inactivity that Haggai was sent to address; it was a matter of right priorities! The people were so busy doing the things that pleased them that they had no time left to do what was pleasing to God. As a result of their persistent procrastination, when it came to caring for God's house, the people were experiencing a "not enough" problem. Stop for a minute and ask yourself, *Is busyness the thing that is keeping me from taking care of the business that is important to God?* Explain your answer.

_____

_____

_____

_____

_____

In verses 5-6, God invites His people to give careful thought to their errant ways. He then gives them five specific examples of the way their refusal to care for His Temple is being manifested in their lives. Using verses 5-6, complete the following sentences:

You . . .	But . . .
Have planted much	
Eat	
Drink	
Put on clothes	
Earn wages	

Certainly, there is nothing wrong with planting, eating, drinking, putting on clothes or earning wages. As a matter of fact, all these things are part of God's gracious provision for His people. So, if what the people were doing was not wrong, what was the problem?

_____

_____

_____

Read Haggai 1:9. What were the people expecting?

_____

_____

_____

What did they actually get?

_____

_____

_____

After looking at what the people expected versus what they actually got, ask yourself this question: *Can I pick and choose the aspects of First Place 4 Health that I enjoy doing while ignoring the ones that are hard for me and still expect to receive God's blessing?* Explain your answer.

_____

_____

_____

Once again, if God were speaking to you through Haggai, what might He tell you is the root cause of the "not enough" you are experiencing? What one thing that is important to God might you be neglecting?

_____

_____

_____

Faithful Father, Your rebuke is not pleasant to my ears, yet I know You teach me because You love me. Thank You for sending Your Word to heal me—and to remind me of what is important to You. Amen.

Day 4 — YOUR BODY IS GOD'S HOUSE

Gracious and loving God, I know that I am not my own, for I have been bought at a price: the precious blood of Jesus! Today, I will care for myself because Jesus loved me enough to die for me and because He asks me to care for myself as a reflection of my love for Him. Amen.

Let's examine the Scriptures to see exactly what house it is that we need to be rebuilding. Certainly, giving our time and money to build or maintain the church building in which we worship is a good thing, but if we are neglecting God's primary home, even the time and money we give to help maintain a physical building can be part of our procrastination. Our first stewardship responsibility is caring for our body, because it is God's Temple!

In his speech before the Sanhedrin, Stephen gave a brief history of God's Temple. Read his words in Acts 7:44-50. What important thing do you learn from these verses?

_____

_____

_____

_____

_____

Through the power of the Holy Spirit, God dwells in *human hearts*. Paul, in writing to the Corinthians, makes it very clear where God now dwells. Turn in your Bible to 1 Corinthians 3:16-17. Carefully think about Paul's words, and then answer the following questions. Each time you see the word "you," substitute your name. Now answer the following questions:

Where does God's Spirit live, and why does the Spirit live there?

_____

_____

_____

Why is neglect of God's house displeasing to God?

_____

_____

_____

Who is that Temple?

_____

_____

_____

How does 1 Corinthians 3:16-17 correspond with Haggai's warning to ancient Israel?

_____

_____

_____

_____

Your body is a precious gift from God, and He has entrusted you with its care. Practicing a healthy lifestyle is your first stewardship responsibility. Even though you may be busy doing lots of other things, it is important that you do not neglect your primary responsibility: to care for God's house. What can you do today to bring any priorities that might be out of balance back in line with God's priorities for your life?

_____

_____

_____

_____

Father, it is beyond my comprehension that the Holy Spirit would take up residence in my humble home. Help me lovingly care for my body because it belongs to You and You have entrusted me with the awesome responsibility of caring for Your Temple.

Day 5 — SWING INTO ACTION

My faithful Father, I am confident that You will give me everything I need to do the work You have put before me. Thank You for giving me the desire to strengthen my body as part of Your gracious provision. Amen.

As we have seen in prior weeks of this study, God never presents us with a problem without also providing a solution. He does not expect us to play 20 Questions or live in confusion and uncertainty. Jesus Christ came so that we could know the truth that would set us free (see John 8:32). Just as soon as God confronted His people with their sin, He quickly told them what they needed to do to become objects of His blessing. Read Haggai 1:7-8. In your own words, write what God told His people they needed to do:

_____

_____

_____

_____

Why is God asking His people to do this work?

"So that I may _____ _____ in it and be _____,"
says the LORD (Haggai 1:8).

In this same verse, what does God tell the people they are to do?

"Go up into the _____ and _____ down
_____."

What does this command imply?

_____

_____

_____

This will be difficult and time-consuming labor—hard physical work that will take planning and preparation. Given this, would the people have been able to do what God commanded them to do and still "do their own thing"? Why or why not?

_____

_____

_____

If God were to give you a major rebuilding project like this, what would you need to eliminate from your life in order to be obedient? (As you ponder this question, remember that God will not ask you to neglect any of His other commandments—things like working to support yourself or care for your family—to comply with His wishes. So it is not the basic things that sustain your life that you might need to abandon. God never asks anything of you unless He knows you are capable of doing it!)

_____

_____

_____

Before we actually begin the physical work, we will need to carefully plan our work so that we will not not be counterproductive in our efforts. But planning alone is not enough. We must turn that plan into action. Someone once said that we must "plan our work and work our plan." How is keeping an accurate record of our daily activities part of planning our work and working our plan?

_____

_____

_____

Are you planning your work and working your plan when it comes to taking care of your body? If not, why not?

_____

_____

_____

_____

> *O Lord, what You ask me to do is not too difficult or beyond my reach.*
> *Help me to diligently obey Your clear command that I care for my body,*
> *because it is Your dwelling place (see Deuteronomy 30:11). Amen.*

Day 6

REFLECTION AND APPLICATION

Lord God, today I commit my plans to You, confident that as I do Your will,
You will bless the work of my hands. I realize that learning Your Word at a
heart level takes work and commitment. With Your help, I will devote
myself to learning and applying Your Word to my life. Amen.

Learning takes place on six levels, beginning with simple recall or recognition of facts and going to the highest level of cognition, which is assimilating information so that it becomes part of our being and belief system. When the apostle Paul asked the piercing question, "Do you not know that your body is a temple of the Holy Spirit?"(1 Corinthians 6:19), he was not asking his readers if they could repeat that verse from memory. He was asking whether or not the surface knowledge had penetrated their being so that the words made a difference in their belief systems and behavior.

It is one thing to repeat a series of words from rote memory; it is another to have the ability to evaluate those words so that they can be compared, defended, valued, acted upon and used as a basis for personal faith. Paul knew that his readers had what we refer to as "head knowledge." What he wanted to know is whether or not that head knowledge had made the 18-inch drop to the heart and become heart knowledge!

Be challenged by Paul's words today: "Do you not know that your body is a temple of the Holy Spirit?" Allow that knowledge to become part of your belief system and behavior.

List five things you learned from this week's lesson that will help you live in a way that reflects the truth that God's Holy Spirit lives inside your heart and mind and that you are committed to caring for your body because He cares for you.

1. _____
2. _____
3. _____
4. _____
5. _____

Loving Lord, I do know that my body is a temple of Your Holy Spirit. Help me apply that knowledge to my life so that I give You glory in all that I do. Amen.

REFLECTION AND APPLICATION

Day 7

Thank You, gracious God, for Your promise to bless me with Your favor from the moment I commit myself to doing the work that pleases You.

In the beginning stages, restoring God's house can seem like an overwhelming task. Yet we can be encouraged when we remember that God has promised to be with us and to bless us as you do the things that please and honor Him. In Haggai 2:15-19, God asked the people to remember what their lives were like before they began to care for His house as He desired. Recap what God was asking them to remember:

_____
_____
_____
_____

Although there was no seed left in the barns and no fruit on the vines, from that day forward God told His people things would be different. What made the difference (see Haggai 2:18)?

_____

_____

_____

_____

Did the whole project need to be completed before God began to bless the people's efforts? No! From the very day the people began to do what God had asked them to do, the quality of their lives changed! Suddenly, God's disfavor turned into blessing. God instructed His people to remember the day they began to lay brick upon brick, because from that day He would bless them.

When we have our priorities straight and are doing the hard work necessary to rebuild God's house according to His desires, we will be able to celebrate success. Living a life pleasing to God makes every day a joyful celebration!

Sovereign Lord, I want to live a life that brings You pleasure. Help me to do the work that You have set before me today and always. Amen.

Group Prayer Requests

4 first place
health

Today's Date: _____

Name	Request

Results

_____

_____

_____

_____

_____

celebrate
with singing

SCRIPTURE MEMORY VERSE
Speak to one another with psalms, hymns and spiritual songs.
Sing and make music in your heart to the Lord.
EPHESIANS 5:19

When we become a new creation in Christ, all of our attitudes and be-
haviors change! Our mind begins to be renewed as the Holy Spirit in-
fuses us with the mind of Christ. Each day, we are being transformed as
God molds and shapes us into the image of His Son, our Lord and Savior, Jesus Christ. As a result of the process, we are commanded in the
New Testament to speak to others in a different way—a way that reflects
what God has done in us.

Because God has created in us a new heart, He places within us a
new song. Gone are the old songs of self-centeredness; a new melody
lives within. The balance and inner harmony, which at one time eluded
us, is now a daily reality. We are no longer on that emotional roller-
coaster ride that characterized our life before the goodness and kindness of God appeared and saved us. We have much to sing about!

This process does not usually happen in the blink of an eye. Rather,
it is a life-long renewal that begins the moment we accept Jesus Christ
as our Lord and Savior, and it continues until the moment we are taken
up in glory to live with God forever. We go from glory to glory as we
grow in grace and knowledge, and we have countless opportunities to
sing His praises to other members of His Body in the form of psalms,
hymns and spiritual songs.

As the memory verse for this week implies, an act of gratitude to the Lord would be to encourage others and build them up in their faith, even as we allow them to build us up. Hebrews 3:13 tells us that we are to encourage one another daily so that we will not become hardened by sin's deceitfulness. We are to be alert and pay attention to the way we live our lives and not allow ourselves to become stumbling blocks to others. Let us rejoice and sing about what God in Christ Jesus has done for us!

One of the greatest blessings to come out of Jesus' sacrificial death and glorious resurrection is the new position of prominence promised to those who place their trust in Christ. They are now children of God, fellow heirs with Christ, and children of the King! As heirs, they are entitled to His inheritance. But of what exactly does that consist, knowing that Jesus basically died a pauper? He didn't have a home, didn't own any land, had no wife or kids, and was even buried in a borrowed tomb. So if He didn't leave any "earthly" inheritance, what did He leave?

Start a list below of what you believe Christ left for you, and then add to it during the week as you look at a few of the great treasures you've inherited to sing about as a son or daughter of the King.

_____

_____

_____

_____

_____

_____

THE SONG OF HOPE

Day 1

Father in Heaven, inspire me to sing of Your goodness this day and give thanks for Christ in me, the Hope of glory. Amen.

Read Titus 3:7. Notice that as heirs of Christ, we inherit the "hope of eternal life." Sometimes the word "hope" can be unclear depending on how it is used. Many of us look at hope as something that might or might not happen. "I *hope* I get to go on a cruise for my anniversary. I *hope* it doesn't rain today! I *hope* that I get the new position, because I think the interview went really well."

What does hope mean to you? Check all that apply.

__	maybe	__	favorable
__	expectation	__	confidence
__	to anticipate	__	trust
__	faith	__	(other) _____

In the context of Titus 3:7, the phrase "the hope of eternal life" is "the full manifestation and realization of that life, which is already the believer's possession."[1] Simply put, our past has been forgiven, we are living in new life at the present, and we have an even greater life to look forward to in the future.

Eternal life became ours when we received His free offer. It's ours now, and it's still to come.

With that understanding, describe a person's life without Christ as depticted in Titus 3:3.

_____
_____
_____
_____
_____

Continuing in Titus 3, read verses 4-5. If we're not saved because of righteous acts, why and how did God save us?

free mercy
_____
_____
_____

What will a person's life look like after he or she is saved (see vv. 5-8)?

_____

_____

_____

_____

John 17:3 gives one of the clearest meanings of "eternal life" found in the Bible. Write this verse in your own words.

_____

_____

_____

_____

We have to know God and His Son, Jesus Christ. Aren't you thankful for a kind, loving and merciful God who has so graciously given us eternal life to live right now but also to look forward to in the future? What an everlasting inheritance we have in Him!

God, thank You for the gift of Your salvation. Let me never lose sight of the life I have in You now and the hope of the eternal life yet to come. You alone are the Giver of Life. I sing to You with all of my heart!

THE SONG OF THE SON
Day 2

Dear God, give me childlike faith this day to live in reverent awe of who You are, Lord of Lords and King of Kings; and help me to enjoy my place in Your kingdom. Amen.

The memory verse this week draws us to speak to one another about the great things God has done for us. Have you ever thought about what the word "great" means? It's an adjective with synonymous meanings such as "eminent, noble, famous, prominent, royal, widely acclaimed, regal, elevated." These words conjure up images of great importance and influence. As children, we prayed, "God is great, God is good," and we were right in doing so. As children of the King of Kings and Lord of Lords, we've inherited the grandest, most royal Kingdom imaginable.

What have we been rescued from in order to be in the kingdom of the Son (see Colossians 1:13)?

_____

_____

_____

Who can see the kingdom of God (see John 3:3)?

_____ *those who are born again* _____

_____

_____

Throughout Scripture, the Kingdom a believer inherits is described in various ways. Look up the following verses and fill in the blanks.

Psalm 145:13:	_____ kingdom
Matthew 3:2:	kingdom of _____
Matthew 25:34:	your *inheritance*, ___ kingdom
1 Corinthians 15:50:	kingdom of _____
2 Timothy 4:1:	_____ kingdom
2 Timothy 4:18:	_____ kingdom
2 Peter 1:11:	_____ kingdom
Revelation 11:15:	the kingdom of _____ _____ and of his _____

Jesus taught the people on numerous occasions about the kingdom of God through the use of parables. In Luke 13:18-21, He compares the kingdom of God to two objects. Name them.

1. _____ *mustard seed* _____
2. _____ *yeast* _____

What do you think He was trying to teach us about the Kingdom by comparing it to these two objects?

_____

_____

_____

In Luke 17:20-21, we find the Pharisees asking Jesus when the kingdom of God would come. Write Jesus' reply to this question below.

_____

_____

_____

There is much more we could learn about the Kingdom, but let's close today's study with one final verse. Luke 12:32 reveals something about the Father of our Kingdom that we should never forget. Write what that is in the space below, and then spend some time thanking Him for His good pleasure.

_____

_____

_____

Heavenly Father, thank You for allowing me to be a part of Your Son's glorious and mighty Kingdom. May my life be worthy of the inheritance that You have so freely given me.

THE SONG OF THE SPIRIT
Day 3

Dear Father, may I walk fully in Your spirit today, seeking You and depending on Your Holy Spirit to guide me in all truth. Amen.

For most of us, regular deposits into our bank account are a necessity that we look forward to every month. It's our assurance that we'll have the necessary funds to make payments toward our earthly possessions, such as our home, a new car, that special entertainment center, and so forth. It's our hope that one day those items will be ours, paid in full.

A similar transaction has taken place for every child of God. According to Ephesians 1:13-14, the Holy Spirit is the deposit that guarantees our inheritance. Other Bible translations use words such as "pledge," "earnest," "down payment" and "guarantee." So, in other words, the Holy Spirit Himself is a deposit, a down payment and a pledge guaranteeing that we will receive the full inheritance promised us by God. That means we can trust Him to help us in our attempts to live a balanced life today.

To better understand this great promise, take a few minutes to work the puzzle on the following page and place the answers in the appropriate blanks.

Across

1. Our deposit—the promised _____ (Ephesians 1:13).
2. Those guaranteed an inheritance are God's _____ (Ephesians 1:14).
3. The Holy Spirit is a deposit _____ our inheritance (Ephesians 1:14).
4. The Spirit Himself testifies with our spirit that we are God's _____ (Romans 8:16).
5. God made us for this very _____ (2 Corinthians 5:5).
6. The Holy Spirit is a deposit guaranteeing our inheritance until the _____ of those who are God's possession (Ephesians 1:14).
7. We were included in Christ when we heard the word of _____ (Ephesians 1:13).
8. We were marked in Christ when we _____ (Ephesians 1:13).

Down

1. The Holy Spirit is a _____ guaranteeing our inheritance (Ephesians 1:14, *NASB*).
2. We were marked in Him with a _____ (Ephesians 1:13).
3. God has placed all things _____ Christ's feet (Ephesians 1:22).
4. Those who are in the possession of _____ will be redeemed (Ephesians 1:14).
5. The Holy Spirit is a _____ guaranteeing our inheritance (Ephesians 1:14).
6. We were _____ with a seal, the promised Holy Spirit (Ephesians 1:13).

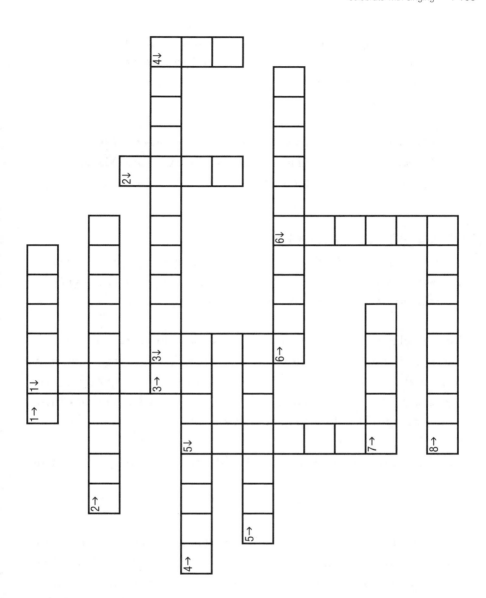

Take time to digest the Scriptures you looked up to answer the puzzle. To really grasp that the Holy Spirit has been given to you and resides in you ought to be a powerful incentive to truly get your body and soul fit for His indwelling.

> *God, continue to reveal to me just what it means to be marked and sealed by Your very Spirit. May I never doubt what You have done in securing my eternal inheritance that is yet to come.*

Day 4 THE SONG OF THE SUFFERING

Father, I pray this day that I may know You, the power of Your resurrection and the fellowship of Your suffering in a way that will do Your great work of transformation in me, for my sake and for Your glory. Amen.

At first glance, most of us would just as soon skip the first part of today's study and focus on the glory part. After all, who in their right mind would want to inherit sufferings? How many of us enjoy singing a funeral dirge? Yet as we look to God's Word today, you will see that Christ's sufferings and His glory go hand in hand.

Read Romans 8:17 and circle true or false for the following statement.

T (F)   Some are called to suffer, while others are called to share His glory.

Although the above statement at times would seem to be true, according to Scripture, all who share in Christ's sufferings will share in His glory. No doubt all of us have experienced or are presently experiencing some degree of suffering. What encouragement and hope does Paul offer in verse 18 of Romans 8?

_____

_____

_____

One obvious misconception among some Christians is that once we give our lives to God and become part of His family, we will have no more worries and everything will be hunky-dory. Nothing could be further from the truth. Look up 2 Corinthians 1:5 and write what Paul said to the church at Corinth.

_____

_____

_____

The same verse in the *New American Standard Bible* reads, "For just as the sufferings of Christ are ours in *abundance*" (emphasis added). Ouch! Face it: we are going to face difficulties and troubles in our life. Knowing this, what can we do to prepare ourselves for those unpleasant times? First Peter 4:12-16 and 5:9-10 offer some of the best advice on dealing with the sufferings that are sure to come our way. How does Peter tell his readers to respond to the trials they are suffering in 1 Peter 4:14?

If you are insulted because of the name of Christ, you are __*blessed*__, for the Spirit of __*glory*__ and of God rests on you.

Are you noticing how many times "glory" is mentioned in relation to "suffering"? What kind of suffering is not included in this blessing (see v. 15)?

_____

_____

_____

You are never alone in the trials and tribulations you go through, even though at the moment you may think you are. Read what Peter said in 1 Peter 5:9. Who besides you is suffering?

_____

_____

_____

In spite of our suffering, we can stand strong knowing that the God of all grace has called us to His _____ _____ in Christ (see v. 10). Now that's a verse worth reading again and making note of the correlation between suffering and glory! We can take heart knowing that our Savior understands all that we go through because of the prophesied sufferings and glories that He himself would experience (see 1 Peter 1:10-11).

> *Almighty God, You truly understand the significance of the sufferings and the glories that I will inherit. Help me accept the bad along with the good and sing Your praises regardless of my circumstances. Amen.*

Day 5 — A SONG OF BLESSING

Dear God, You give and take away. May I say with all my heart, "Blessed be Your name"; name above all names, the name that gives hope and life. In Your name I will live this day. Amen.

On Day 2 of this week, we looked briefly at the great things worth making music about in our hearts. Today, we will focus on the things that bring joy as we look at yet another great thing the Lord has done for us by calling us to receive and to be a blessing. When we take the time to "Speak to one another with psalms, hymns and spiritual songs," we are actually imparting a blessing on someone.

Before you get into the Scripture, look at some of the ways *Webster's New World Dictionary* defines the word "blessing":

> **Blessing:** A statement of divine favor; an invoking of divine favor; the gift of divine favor; hence, a wish for prosperity, success, etc.; anything that gives happiness or prevents misfortune.

Going a step further, the Greek word for "blessing," *eulogia*, can mean a blessing as a benefit—bestowed by God or Christ. It carries with it the idea of bounty or bountifully, in order that blessed influence might be felt.[2] With that in mind, read Genesis 12:2-3 and note how many times the word "bless," "blessed" or "blessing" is used:

I will make you into a great nation and I will _____ you,

I will make your name great, and you will be a _____.

I will _____ those who _____ you, and whoever curses you I will curse;

and all people on earth will be _____ through you.

This passage is a promise made by God to Abram (aka Abraham), and what a powerful promise it is. Not only does God say that He is going to bless Abraham, but He also says that Abraham will be a blessing and the peoples on the earth will be blessed through him. Jump forward to Hebrews 6:13-15. How did Abraham receive what was promised (see v. 15)?

_____

_____

_____

_____

What does Peter say God's chosen people will inherit in 1 Peter 3:8-9?

_____

_____

_____

_____

According to those same verses, how should the Christian who inherits this blessing be living?

_____

_____

_____

_____

Begin making a list of the blessings you consider to be a part of what God has promised. To broaden your thinking, read Ephesians 1:3 and 2:6 before you begin.

Blessings I have received	Future blessings

Abraham's blessings included being the father of a great nation, having wealth and enjoying prosperity. He was even called God's friend (see James 2:23)! It doesn't get much better than that. Just as God promised to bless Abraham, He has promised that we will inherit a blessing. Some of those blessings we are receiving now, but the greatest blessing of our future home with Him is one for which we will have to patiently wait.

God, remind me to share the blessing of You with others so that they, too, may inherit all that You have in store for them. Blessed be Your name!

Day 6 — REFLECTION AND APPLICATION

Lord, Your Word is truth. May I speak truth in love to all who come across my path. May my conversations be seasoned with salt and filled with light.

First Corinthians 13:4-7 helps us learn how to speak God's native language: the language of love. After a long list of "love does not," Paul tells us there are four things that love always does: "Love always protects, always trusts, always hopes, always perseveres" (v. 7). Each of these aspects of love plays a vital role in our success. Beside each listing, write how these four items are part of the way we are to take care of ourselves as part of the First Place 4 Health program.

Love always protects   _____

Love always trusts   _____

Love always hopes   _____

Love always perseveres   _____

First Corinthians 13:8 tells us that love never fails. What specific love do you think Paul is speaking of in that statement? (Hint: It is not human love!)

_____

_____

_____

_____

_____

Finally, look at 1 Corinthians 13:13. How are faith, hope and love part of your life? Be prepared to share your answer with your group at the next meeting so they can all benefit from your words.

_____

_____

_____

_____

Almighty God, I can be strong and courageous because You have promised to never leave me nor forsake me. Because of Your goodness and kindness to me, I can be good and kind to others. I know that I can only love because You first loved me. Amen.

Day 7

REFLECTION AND APPLICATION

Father, I thank You that by the power of Your Holy Spirit, You allow me to share my experience, strength and hope with those in need. Amen.

This week's memory verse tells us how we are to speak to one another. We are to speak to our brothers and sisters in Christ with:

_____, _____,

and _____.

Our memory verse also tells us how we are to speak to ourselves!

_____ and make _____ in our _____ to the Lord.

On this day of reflection, you are going to put both of those admonitions into practice. Go to Psalms and pick a psalm (or a portion of a psalm) that you would like to share with someone in your group. This could either be with your prayer partner or someone in the group who is really struggling right now. Write the psalm on a note card and mail it to that person in "secret pal" fashion (without a return address or name).

After you have spoken in this way to another person—in psalms, hymns and spiritual songs—it is time to encourage yourself by singing and making music in your heart to the Lord. Pick a favorite hymn or praise song and sing it to yourself (and to God) as part of your quiet time today. Even if you are not musical, you can sing in your heart, because only God will hear the joyful noise you are making unto Him!

Thank you, Lord, for encouraging me in my faith and asking me to encourage others as well. Today I will sing in the shadow of Your wings.

Notes

1. W. E. Vine, *An Expository Dictionary of New Testament Words* (Old Tappan, NJ: Fleming H. Revell Co., 1966), vol. 2, p. 233.
2. Walter Bauer, *A Greek-English Lexicon of the New Testament and Other Early Christian Literature* (Chicago and London: The University of Chicago Press, 1979), pp. 322-323.

Group Prayer Requests

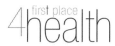

Today's Date: _____9- 11 - 1 4_____

Name	Request
Eugene & Mary Lou	
Shelly Long	
Donna & Jim Fish	
Courtney	
Mary	

Results

_____

_____

_____

_____

_____

celebrate God's goodness

9-18-14

SCRIPTURE MEMORY VERSE
*The LORD has done great things for us,
and we are filled with joy.*
PSALM 126:3

Although our society celebrates many things, in God's kingdom, celebration is always an occasion to remember God's goodness. The memory verse for this week tells us what our proper response should be when we remember this. Write this three-letter word in capital letters in the space below:

J   O   Y

Take this joy with you as you begin your day. Let it color your world and fill you with gratitude for all the good things the Lord has done for you—and promises to continue doing throughout eternity.

Day 1 — REJOICE IN THE LORD

*O Lord God, You have given me all I need to live a life worthy of my calling.
I can rest secure in Your love, no matter my circumstances. Amen.*

When the apostle Paul wrote the epistle to the Christians in Philippi, he was locked in a Roman prison, chained to a guard and living in conditions most of us would consider anything but joyful. Yet even though he was writing from prison, his letter is full of joy. In fact, the words "joy" or "rejoice" are used 14 times in this short epistle! Perhaps the most well-known of all Paul's writings on the subject of joy is found in Philippians 4:4-7. Turn to that passage now as you examine how Paul could be filled with joy, even in the midst of affliction.

Philippians 4:4 begins with a bold declaration:

Rejoice in the _Lord_ _always_.

Those words are the first lesson about the source of our joy. What are we being exhorted to rejoice in?

The Lord is near

Is this rejoicing to be an occasional activity—something we do when our lives are going well? Explain your answer.

Yes I rejoice when things are going well but I pray that I can rejoice in all circumstances

Notice that Paul does not say, "Rejoice in your circumstances!" Often, our circumstances are nothing to rejoice over. In John 16:33, Jesus told His disciples what to expect in this world. Put a marker in the Philippians passage and turn to John 16:33. What does Jesus tell us, His modern-day disciples, to expect?

In this world you will have trouble but God has overcome the world

If you are going to have trouble, how can you take heart? (The last sentence in John 16:33 contains the answer.)

God has overcome the world

Jesus has overcome the world, but we live in that period in salvation history where the fullness of Jesus' victory over sin and death has not yet been fully realized. We live in a "yet, but not yet" world—we know the outcome but still live with tribulation. Our reward is sure, but we will have to wait until Jesus returns to realize it in full measure. Turning back to Philippians 4:4, what do you see Paul doing in the last sentence of the verse?

Rejoice

What does the fact that Paul has repeated his words tell you?

He wants us to know He means what He says

Rejoicing is not an option for those who desire to live a life pleasing to God. Rejoicing is part of the very fiber of our being! Spend the rest of your quiet time today rejoicing in God's goodness. You might want to use this week's memory verse as the springboard for your joyful praise!

> O Lord God, You have done great things for me. Today I will respond
> to Your love and mercy by rejoicing in Your love. Amen.

CELEBRATE GOD'S PRESENCE

Day 2

Gracious God, You have promised to never abandon me or forsake me.
You have promised to always be near; to never leave me to face my
problems, even those of my own making, by myself. I rejoice in Your love.

Yesterday, we began to examine Philippians 4:4-7 to determine how the apostle Paul could be joyful even though he was locked in a Roman jail while writing those words. Summarize what you learned yesterday.

We should & can rejoice in all circumstances if we look for the good

In Philippians 4:5, Paul begins to give the reason we can be joyful even in affliction. But before telling us how to rejoice, he begins by telling us how we should act toward others as a result of our determination to rejoice always. What does the first sentence of Philippians 4:5 tell us to do?

Let your gentleness be evident to all.

According to Philippians 4:5, what people are you to be gentle toward? Think of all the people you meet during the course of a day. Name at least one person who could benefit from your "gentleness." What would that gentleness look like?

everyone
I should check on my friend Lyene more often.

The word "all," like "always," leaves no room for exception! We are to let our gentleness be known to all. How is gentleness the result of rejoicing always?

I we are rejoicing we are more at ease with everything

In the second half of Philippians 4:5, Paul tells us the secret that allows us to be gentle with others, even when we are in difficult circumstances. What does Paul tells us in the last sentence of Philippians 4:5?

The Lord is near.

Turn in your Bible to Joshua 1:9. What did the Lord tell Joshua about being strong and courageous?

Do not be discouraged for the Lord will be with you wherever you go.

How does being gentle to all require strength and courage?

Some people are not easy to be gentle to

How can Philippians 4:5 help you be joyful, even when your patience and tolerance are running at a low ebb because you are trying to make important changes in your life?

Remember the Lord is near

Lord God, all too often I forget that You are near, ready to help me and guide me if I will only ask for Your help. Today I will choose to rejoice, not because my circumstances are ideal but because You are near. Amen.

ANXIOUS ABOUT NOTHING

Day 3

Father God, I often worry and fret rather than rejoice in Your presence and Your love. Help me to never question Your wisdom or spend my time and energy in anxiety and uncertainty. Amen.

If we were asked to describe the opposite of rejoicing, our first inclination might be to say "sadness." But the apostle Paul tells us it is something else. Turn in your Bible to Philippians 4:6 and read what Paul tells us not to do if we are going to rejoice always. What did you discover?

Do not be anxious

Once again, the apostle Paul is very clear about what we are not to be anxious about. According to Philippians 4:6, is anxiety ever acceptable? Explain your answer.

in everything by prayer

In your own words, explain how anxiety is the opposite of rejoicing because the Lord is near.

we are gentle in rejoicing
we are nervous in anxiety

Anxiety has a compound effect. What are we who are traveling the First Place 4 Health journey prone to do when we are anxious?

eat

Instead of turning to comfort food to settle our anxious spirit, the apostle Paul tells us to do something else. What does he say to do, and when are we to do it?

prayer, thanksgiving

Are there any exceptions to Paul's admonition to present our requests to God? (What word does Paul use in Philippians 4:6 that gives you the answer to this question?)

every thing

"Always," "all," "nothing," "everything"! Paul leaves no wiggle room for doing things our way—for falling back into old anxious ways! Rather than being anxious, we are to present our prayers and petitions to

God. According to Philippians 4:6, how are we to present our requests to God?

but in every thing, by prayer & petition with thanksgiving present your request to God.

How can this week's memory verse be used to present your prayers and petitions to God with thanksgiving?

The Lord has done great things and we are filled will joy

Write a prayer to God in the space below, incorporating the thoughts of Psalm 126:3 into your petition.

Dear God as you have given me time to see all of the things I am to to rejoice in, let me have a gentle and rejoiceful day

Lord, You have done great things for me. Even as I present my petitions to You today, I can rejoice and be thankful, for I know You never change. Your mercies are new every morning and Your faithfulness is great.

PRAYER PRODUCES PEACE

Day 4

Lord, I do not always comprehend Your ways, but today I choose to trust in You. Please give me Your peace and guide my heart and my mind. Amen.

God's peace will guard your heart and your mind! How is this guarding of your heart and mind one of the ways the Lord has been good to you? Explain your answer.

God makes me sat back & see the good in what He does even though I don't see it at the time

Yesterday, we discussed the universal antidote to anxiety: rejoicing in prayer! Remembering what you learned, how are you to present your requests to God, and when are you to do so? List at least three things you learned about prayer yesterday (or had reinforced if you are already a seasoned prayer warrior).

1. _the Lord is always there & hears_
2. _our prayers so that we don't have_
3. _to become anxious._

Philippians 4:7 gives us the predictable results of our prayer and petitions that are presented to God with thanksgiving. What is this predictable result?

the peace of God will guard our hearts & minds in Jesus Christ.

Interestingly, Paul does not say that we will get what we have asked for, he just says we will have peace! And not just any peace! What type of peace will prayer produce?

The peace of God

How is the peace that Paul is talking about the same kind that is described in Proverbs 3:5-6?

Proverbs 3:5-6 tells you that you are to trust in the Lord rather than leaning on your own _understanding._

Philippians 4:7 says that you will have peace that transcends all _understanding_

What do these verses (Proverbs 3:5-6 and Philippians 4:7) tell us about our ability to comprehend God's ways?

we can not know Gods ways but we can have peace that He knows the way

Fortunately, our inability to understand God's ways does not keep God from acting in ways that we don't understand! How is God asking you to trust in Him rather than relying on your own understanding?

pray

When we don't understand God's ways, are we to become anxious and afraid? If not, what are we to do instead? (Combine what you have learned in Philippians 4:4-7 with Proverbs 3:5-6 in your answer.)

pray & have peace that God hears.

What will God's peace do that the peace offered by the philosophies of this world can't possibly do? (The answer is found in the last sentence of Philippians 4:7.)

the peace of God will guard our hearts & minds

God's peace will guard your heart and your mind! How is this guarding of your heart and mind one of the ways the Lord has been good to you? Explain your answer.

Thank You, Lord God, for peace that passes understanding. Thank You that I can rejoice in You, no matter what my circumstances. Today I will rejoice in Your love. Amen.

Day 5

THINK ABOUT THESE THINGS

Lord, today I ask that You would help me to focus on those things that are from You and present my cares to You so that I will be anxious in nothing.

The apostle Paul ends his exhortation to "rejoice in the Lord always" by giving some specific instructions about what we are to think about and what we are to dwell on. The list of these things appears below. Next to each "whatever," list one way you are seeking to follow that instruction. For instance, "whatever is true" could be manifesting in your life if you are studying God's Word and applying the truths you find to your life.

Whatever is . . .	How this "whatever" is being manifested in my life
True	*I am studying God's Word and applying the truths I find for healthy living.*
Noble	
Right	
Pure	
Lovely	
Admirable	
Excellent	
Praiseworthy	

If you were to dwell on these "whatevers," how might you be better equipped to rejoice always?

Pray & ask God to help me with these cares & concerns

How would you be better able to display gentleness to all?

Don't always look for my way

How would your thoughts help you to be anxious for nothing?

know that in His timing God will answer

How would you be more willing to present everything to God in prayer and petition with thanksgiving?

by knowing He is always near

Of all the things Paul has told us to do in Philippians 4:4-8, which will be most difficult for you to incorporate into your life?

do not be anxious

What one thing can you do today to begin to make this change, even though it will be difficult?

Merciful Father, I know You do not ask me to do anything that is too difficult or beyond my reach. Today I will present my petitions to You with thanksgiving, knowing that Your peace will transcend my understanding.

Day 6

REFLECTION AND APPLICATION

O God of hope, You fill me with joy and peace as I trust in You. Today, I will rejoice in Your love and goodness and meditate on Your kindness, compassion and tender mercy. Amen.

The memory verse for this week was one of the marching cadences used by the singers in ancient Israel who marched into battle in front of the fighting men. Say the verse over in your mind and picture the singers marching ahead of the army to the beat of these words: "The Lord has done great things for us. And we are filled with joy."

Today, you will use that marching cadence during your exercise time. Put on your walking shoes and let this psalm of praise fill your heart as you walk in rhythm to the words you are saying in your mind. As you say these words over and over again, remember that the Lord is near. And not only is He near, but He is the same yesterday, today and forever. The same God who marched into battle with the ancient Israelites is marching in step with you!

When you have completed your walk, take a few minutes to record the thoughts and images that walking in sync with the words of this week's memory verse brought up for you. Could you picture yourself marching alongside David and Daniel, Samuel and Moses, Peter and Paul, James and John? Could you feel the presence of the Lord Himself filling your heart and mind with His peace—a peace that transcends your understanding? End your writing with a joyful affirmation that the Lord has done great things for you, and then march into the day with joy.

Gracious God, I know that I am surrounded by a great cloud of witnesses (see Hebrews 12:1). Thank You for allowing me to march in Your joyful procession with those who have gone before me. Amen.

REFLECTION AND APPLICATION

You have done such great things for me, O Lord. Today I will respond by trusting Your goodness and grace enough to let go of my painful past. Amen.

Celebrate Success is about remembering the good things God has done for us and responding to His goodness by living a life worthy of our calling in Jesus Christ. Today, we will look at God's goodness as a personal invitation to do the following:

- Let Jesus do for you what He has done for so many others before you.
- Love again, after your love has been rejected and you are tempted to hate.
- Hope again, after your hope has been dashed to pieces and you are tempted to despair.
- Believe again, after your belief has been shaken and you are tempted to doubt.
- Pick up the broken pieces and start again, after discouragement has crushed you and you are ready to quit.
- Affirm that Jesus has defeated evil, and so will you.
- Accept the good news that Jesus is alive and active in your world, ready to work miracles for you, if you but let Him.

As you read over this list of invitations, pick the two that you feel are beckoning to you today in a special way. Write an R.S.V.P. to God in response to His personal invitation to you. In the response, affirm your confidence that He is able to accomplish this thing for you and your willingness to respond to His generous offer by doing everything He tells you to do.

You, O Lord, have done great things for me, and I am filled with joy.

Group Prayer Requests

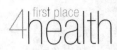

Today's Date: _____

Name	Request
Mary Lou & Eugene	
Lyane	
Donna & Jim Fisk	
Shelly Long	
Judy Hall	
Lori	

Results

_____

_____

_____

_____

_____

celebrate
worship

9-25-'14

SCRIPTURE MEMORY VERSE
*Come, let us bow down in worship,
let us kneel before the LORD our Maker.*
PSALM 95:6

Earlier in this study, you considered what a topsy-turvy world we all live in and how Jesus, our Savior, came to turn the world upside down as He proclaimed the good news of the kingdom of God. No wonder Romans 12:2 warns us against the dangers of letting the world squeeze us into its mold! And perhaps nowhere is the difference between the thoughts of the world and the truth of God's Word more evident than the subject of celebration.

The world encourages us to use celebration as an opportunity to indulge our sinful nature and forget that God's grace demands an appropriate response. For those who have been redeemed by God's grace, celebration is an occasion to remember the good things our gracious Lord has done for us, things that fill us with joy. Ephesians 2:10 tells us that we are God's workmanship, "created in Christ Jesus to do good works, which God prepared in advance for us to do." God paid a very high price to redeem us from a life of sin and death. Write the words of John 3:16 below to remind yourself of the price paid for your freedom:

For God so loved the world that he gave His only Son that whosoever believes in Him shall not perish, but have everlasting life
eternal

Scripture is very clear that there is absolutely nothing we can do to earn God's love and unmerited favor. We are saved by God's grace and God's grace alone. However, having been brought into the family of God through belief in Jesus Christ, we must live as obedient children who earnestly desire to do the will of God. As you will learn in this week's lessons, everything that acknowledges God as your Maker is an opportunity to worship God and give Him the glory and honor He deserves.

Day 1 — WORSHIP ACKNOWLEDGES LORDSHIP

Gracious God, so often I look at the mundane events of my life as trivial when, in fact, they are occasions to worship You in spirit and in truth. Today I will worship You by giving You glory in all that I do. Amen.

Most of us are familiar with the story of how the Lord used Moses to deliver His chosen people from the cruel oppression of Pharaoh. With great displays of power, God's stretched out His hand and led His people out of bondage. However, few of us realize why the Lord wanted Moses to lead the children of God out of Egypt. Exodus 8:1 tells us the reason. Turn in your Bible to that verse and fill in the missing words:

This is what the LORD says: "_let_ my _people_ go, so that they may _worship_ me."

Often, we think of worship as that hour or so we spend each week in church. And, certainly, when we join with our brothers and sisters in Christ to praise and thank God, it is an act of worship. But that is not the only time that we are called to worship God.

Our word "worship" is actually a combination of two words, "worth" and "ship," and by putting those two words together, we get the true essence of the word "worship." When we give God His worth, (what is due Him) by giving Him thanks and praise, every activity we engage in becomes an act of worship.

Two other words that are often combined with the word "ship" help us better understand the concept of worship. Look up the following words in a dictionary and write out their meanings:

Kingship: _a person prominent in their class_

Lordship: _the domaine of a Lord_

Now add together the three "ship" words: "worship," "kingship" and "lordship":

When we _worship_ God, we are acknowledging His _prominence_ and His _domain_ in our life!

In the First Place 4 Health program, you are learning to lead a healthier lifestyle so that you can really begin to worship God as He desires that you worship Him!

O Lord God Almighty, You are indeed worthy of all glory, all honor and all praise. Today I will worship You by caring for the body You created. When I do the things that please You, I am worshiping You. Amen.

A FESTIVAL TO THE LORD

Day 2

O Lord, I confess that I am not my own. I was bought with a price. In gratitude, I will worship You by putting You first in all things. Amen.

What do you think of when you hear the word "festival"?

a celebration with a group of people

A dictionary will tell you that "festival" can mean different things:

1. A time or a day of feasting or celebration; esp. a periodic religious celebration
2. A celebration, entertainment or series of performances of a certain kind, often held periodically
3. Merrymaking, festivity

Which of those three definitions most closely matches what you wrote as your definition of the word "festival," and why?

_②_

Turn to Exodus 10:7-9 and see which definition most closely describes God's definition of a festival. How did Moses use the word "festival" in this passage?

everyone was to go & celebrate the Lord

Still looking at Exodus 10:7-9, when Pharaoh asked Moses exactly who would be going out to worship the Lord, what was Moses' reply?

all people & animals

What does that statement tell you about the importance of family worship (which in ancient Israel also included the animals!) in God's design for celebrating a festival to the Lord?

it is important to all come together

How can you teach your family members to live responsibly before God? (Remember that actions speak louder than words!)

by bringing together with us as we worship

List one thing you will do today to worship God and celebrate His goodness to you through the new freedom you have found in Him.

pray for all my hurting friends & take care of my body.

O Lord my Maker, when I am obedient to Your command that tells me to give glory to You in all that I do, I am bowing down to worship You. Today I will acknowledge Your Lordship in my life, as my creator, sustainer and redeemer. Amen.

WORSHIPING OUR MAKER — Day 3

I praise You, my Maker, because I am fearfully and wonderfully made. You fashioned me to do the work You call me to do. Help me to worship You through diligent care of Your creation. Amen.

The memory verse this week is Psalm 95:6. If you are able to do so, write the verse from memory. (If you haven't memorized it yet, look back at the beginning of this week and write it in the space below.)

Come, let us bow down in worship. Let us kneel before the Lord our Maker.

You might also want to write this verse on a 3x5 card and carry it with you throughout the day. You can use those times when you are waiting in line, stuck in traffic or taking a break from your busy activities to hide God's Word in your heart—which is another form of worship. Look at the words you just wrote. We are to kneel before the _Lord_ our _Maker_. Ephesians 2:10 tells us that we are God's handiwork, created by Him to achieve His plan and purpose. Not only did God make us, but He also purposefully created us according to His design.

The idea that God has crafted us to His exact specifications is found throughout Scripture. Psalm 139:13-15 also speaks eloquently about God our Maker. What phrases in that passage are words we associate with crafting?

> You _knit_ me together in my mother's womb (see v. 13).
> When I was _woven_ together in the depths of the earth (see v. 15).

What comes to mind when you think of God knitting and weaving you together according to His pattern for your life? As you have done in previous studies, use your imagination as you picture God shaping and reshaping you according to His plan for your life.

He has had to reshape me to His design several times

Psalm 139:14 gives our appropriate response: We are to praise God and consider His handiwork wonderful. Do you think of your body as a wonderful masterpiece, fashioned by the Maker of heaven and earth? If not, explain why not. If yes, tell what you are doing to preserve God's special creation called you.

The prophets Isaiah and Jeremiah used another crafting term to describe God, our Maker. Turn to Jeremiah 18:6 to see the analogy Jeremiah uses. What relationship did you discover?

like clay in the hands of the potter

Now turn to Isaiah 29:16. In this verse, Isaiah uses the analogy of the potter and clay to discuss our relationship with God. Paraphrase the question that he asks in your own words, being sure to note the upside-down, topsy-turvy way that we often relate to our Maker.

we are like clay in the hands of the Lord. He will form us

Isaiah 64:8 gives three examples of our relationship to God. Complete the list below by filling in the spaces. Two of the relationships are implied by the text.

He is . . .	We are . . .
The Father	His _possible_
The Potter	The _clay_
The _Lord_	The work of His hands

How might the analogy of the artisan and the work of His hands have a personal application to how God is fashioning you?

_____
_____
_____
_____

Are you humbly submitting to God's plan and purpose for you by doing all you can to protect and cherish His handiwork? Explain your answer.

_____
_____
_____
_____

O Lord, You are the potter and I am the clay. I have no reason to question what You are doing in my life.

Day 4 AN INVITATION TO A CELEBRATION

O Lord, I want to do what You ask of me. Help me to follow after You instead of always seeking greener pastures—pastures where I can do what I want to do rather than following Your lead. Amen.

This week's memory verse comes from Psalm 95, which begins with the invitation: "Come." Read verses 1 and 2 of Psalm 95 and summarize what you are being invited to do by the opening words of this psalm:

Come & be joyful
_____
_____
_____

What words are used in Psalm 95:1-2 that lead you to believe this is a grand celebration?

sing, shout, joy, music & songs

In our memory verse, God is referred to as "our Maker." What word does Psalm 95:1 use to describe the Lord?

the Rock of our salvation

What mental image comes up for you when you see this word being used to describe God? Why is this image a reason to sing for joy and shout aloud?

a solid farm

Psalm 95:3-5 tells us about some of the other things God that has made. What word in verse 5 also speaks of craftsmanship?

His hands formed

After inviting us to bow down in worship and kneel before the Lord our Maker in verse 6, the psalmist tells us another truth about God in verse 7. Not only is God our Maker, but He is our Shepherd. Although the word "shepherd" is not used in this verse, what words does the psalmist use to tell us that the Lord is our Shepherd?

we are the people of His flock

In addition to being our Maker, God is also our Sustainer—the One who cares for us by providing for us and protecting us from savage beasts. As the sheep who live in the Good Shepherd's pasture, what is our responsibility?

obey the Good Shepard

At the end of verse 7, the psalmist writes, "Today, if you hear his voice." After this admonishment to hear God's voice, we are warned against hardening our hearts. Psalm 95:8 recalls a time when the Israelites quarreled with God by questioning His providential care. What does verse 9 say they did?

Your fathers _tested_ and _tried_ me, though they had seen what I did.

Would you say that Jesus Christ has top billing in your life? When it comes to the practical application of God's Word, have you ever hardened your heart and not want to do what He said? (Jesus asked this same question in Luke 6:46.) If so, describe that time.

How is this question applicable to your willingness to consistently apply the principles of healthy living on a daily basis?

Today, Gracious God, I will boast because the Lord is my Shepherd. As a sheep in Your pasture, I shall not want. You will lead me and guide me into right paths. Thank You for Your goodness and love. Amen.

HUMBLE CELEBRATION

Day 5

Gracious God, I accept Your invitation to come and celebrate by giving You Your rightful place as the Lord of my life. Because You are my Lord, I can rejoice and be glad in You. Amen.

Scripture tells us about a celebration held to honor King Herod's birthday. This account is recorded in both Matthew and Mark. Turn in your Bible to Mark 6:21-24. What happened as a result of Herod's desire to impress those in attendance at his lavish birthday bash?

he was forced to behead John

Now turn to Matthew 14:3-4. Why did Herod have John the Baptist thrown into prison?

because of his brother Phillips wife Herodias

Self-indulgence takes many forms. One of Herod's sins was covetousness. He wanted his brother's wife! Given the fact that he summoned a young girl to dance for the crowd, what can we surmise might have been another of Herod's self-gratification sins?

sex

Sexual sins are rampant in our society, even among those who regularly attend church. What other self-indulgent sin is prevalent in today's society but is often seen as socially acceptable behavior?

same self scarings

Overeating is serious to God, because in His eyes, overeating is excess. Scripture tells us that all the sins of excess can be lumped together under one category: indulging the flesh. How are you working to address this age-old problem of "indulging the flesh?" (Remember that "excess" affects your entire being, not just the way you eat.)

Physical excess _trying to slow down_

Mental excess _____

Emotional excess _____

Spiritual excess _____

Turn to Romans 13:14. Because we have been chosen to be God's humble people, clothed with Christ, what are we not to do?

do not gratify the desires of a sinful nature

What does 2 Corinthians 10:5 tell us we are to do about thoughts that do not reinforce our commitment to healthful eating?

Demolish then

How is refusing to indulge the flesh worshiping God, your Maker?

God wants us to have a healthy body

List one thing you need to stop doing today so that you can humbly bow before the Lord your God and join in the humble celebration that puts Christ first in all things.

watch how much I eat.

Today, O Lord, I will bring my thoughts captive to Christ and not even think about how to satisfy the desires of my sinful nature. It is my desire to worship You in all I say and do. Amen.

REFLECTION AND APPLICATION

Day
6

I will rejoice in You, my Maker. I will be glad in my King and sing praises to Your holy name. I will bow down and worship You because You are the Lord of my life. Amen.

Psalm 95:1-3 invites us, "Come, let us sing for joy to the LORD; let us shout aloud to the Rock of our salvation. Let us come before him with thanksgiving and extol him with music and song. For the LORD is the great God, the great King above all gods."

Today, instead of sitting down and reading your lesson, you are going to do a meditation in motion! Before you begin, recall one of your favorite praise songs—one you can sing from memory. (If you're not musically inclined, the music CD in the back of this book is perfect for today's assignment.)

As you begin to sing God's praise, move your feet in step with the rhythm of the music (swinging your arms in sync with your stride will increase the benefits of this meditation in motion). Even if you are in a small space, you can walk in place and enjoy worshiping your Maker by exercising the wonderful body He has crafted especially for you! Your spirits will be lifted and your body energized when you celebrate God's goodness in song.

After you have finished this exercise, carry the songs you used in this meditation time with you throughout the day. God indwells the praises of His people. When you are extolling the Lord with music and a song in your heart, even the most menial tasks will become a reason for celebration. Come, let us sing for joy to the Lord!

> *How good it is to sing praises to You, O God! How good it is to exercise the wonderfully made body You have given me as I sing to You! Thank You for giving me the opportunity to worship You in this way. Amen.*

Day
7
REFLECTION AND APPLICATION

Gracious God, I am Your handiwork, created and equipped so that I can accomplish the plans You have for me. Thank You for giving me feet to follow You in obedience to Your invitation to worship You. Amen.

Our memory verse for this week invites us to bow down in worship and kneel before the Lord our Maker. Although most of us no longer bow and kneel as part of our worship experience, we are still called to worship God with our bodies, not just our spirits. In Romans 12:1, Paul boldly tells us to offer our bodies as living sacrifices, holy and pleasing to God—which is our spiritual worship.

During your reflection time today, you will learn a type of whole-body prayer that will allow you to worship God with your body in a practical way. As you begin this mini-meditation, sit in a comfortable position in a place where there are no outside distractions. Now focus your attention and begin to picture your prayer as a movement that proceeds through your body, beginning with your mind. (It might help to read through the bulleted list below before you begin so that the words and sensations can flow through your body without the need to stop and read the next line.)

As you begin, picture the various parts of your body worshiping in this way:

- Your **mind** praying as you bring your ideas and thoughts into conformity with God's Word.
- Your **lips** praying as you speak to God in audible words.
- Your **eyes** praying when you visualize your requests and see the truth of God's Word.
- Your **ears** praying as you hear God speaking to you.
- Your **heart** praying through your feelings and emotions as you respond to God's love.
- Your **arms** praying as they extend in praise.
- Your **hands** praying as you reach out to minister to others in God's name.
- Your **feet** praying when you respond in obedience to His call, "Follow me."

If there are other body parts that you would like to add to this list, feel free to do so! When you have completed this prayer time, record what it felt like to worship God with your body in your prayer journal.

O Lord, I am Your handiwork, created and equipped so that I can accomplish the plans You have for me. Thank You for giving me lips to praise Your name. Thank You for giving me eyes to see You. Thank You for giving me ears to hear the truth of Your Word.

Group Prayer Requests

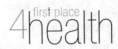

Today's Date: _____

Name	Request

Results

_____

_____

_____

_____

_____

celebrate
stillness

SCRIPTURE MEMORY VERSE
*Be still, and know that I am God;
I will be exalted among the nations,
I will be exalted in the earth.*
PSALM 46:10

God's Word to us is clear. His message echoes in the pages of Scripture and is repeated over and over again lest we miss the importance of what the Mighty One is asking us to do. "Be still and know that I am God." "Be still before the Lord." "The Lord will fight for you; you need only to be still."

Yet even though God's words are unmistakably clear, stillness is a spiritual practice that few of us have mastered—even those of us who desire to give God first place in all things. Give us a busy work task or a project and a deadline and we will spend time and energy and effort to accomplish—and accomplish well—the task at hand. But ask us to "be still and know," and we don't have a clue where to begin. Perhaps one of the problems we encounter when we begin to contemplate stillness is that we all too often confuse stillness with inactivity—with nothingness—when in fact stillness is perhaps the most difficult work we will ever be asked to do!

During the course of this study, you have learned many new things that have put you on the path to success. You have learned how success in First Place 4 Health radically differs from the success celebrated by the world and the culture we live in. You have seen how Jesus came to turn things upside down and introduce you to a new way—a better way. You have been equipped and empowered to make the better choice—the choice that leads to health, balance, inner wholeness and peace with God. Now it is time for you to be still and allow the Holy Spirit to apply what you have learned so that the Word that has been planted in your heart and mind can germinate, sprout, flourish and bear abundant fruit.

Day 1 — QUIETNESS AND TRUST

O Lord God, You call me to be still before You. You tell me that my help comes in quietness and trust, not in my ability to do things in my own strength and power. Thank You, merciful Savior, for teaching me the way You want me to be before You. Amen.

Although God continually asks His people to be still, throughout salvation history, God's people have chosen to ignore God's words and turn instead to their own devices. The prophet Isaiah called this reliance on self "obstinacy." In today's language, we might use the words "hardheaded," "stubborn" or "difficult to control." For an example of God's description of obstinate, turn in your Bible to Psalm 32:9 and write what God is telling His people in this verse.

_____

_____

_____

_____

How have you been stubborn when it comes to obeying the Lord's Word when it tells you to be still and rely on His strength and power rather than your ability to take matters into your own hands?

_____

_____

_____

_____

How is being still before the Lord part of caring for your "Temple"?

_____

_____

_____

_____

Turn in your Bible to Isaiah 30:15-18. Take note of exactly who it is who is speaking in this passage—although the words came from Isaiah's pen, he was only the scribe who put those words on paper. What does Isaiah tell us the Lord longs to do?

_____

_____

_____

_____

According to Isaiah 30:18, who are the ones the Lord blesses?

_____

_____

_____

What is God's message to His people in Isaiah 30:15? As you read this passage, don't be confused by the word "salvation." Isaiah was not talking about eternal salvation but rather about deliverance from the enemies that were warring against the nation of Israel. Even those of us who are saved by the grace of Jesus Christ need to practice repentance, rest, quietness and trust, for we are still living in an enemy-infested land!

_____

_____

_____

What does God say His people were refusing to do in the last part of Isaiah 30:15?

_____

_____

_____

Even though God says He longs to be gracious to His people, what were the people saying? (Isaiah 30:16 has the answer.)

_____

_____

_____

Sovereign Lord, the Holy One of Israel, I have heard Your voice today. It is so much easier for me to rely on the swift horses of this world, to use quick-fix schemes that promise swift results, rather than be still before You. Help me to be still before You today. Amen.

Day 2 · THE LORD WILL FIGHT FOR YOU

Merciful Father, You long to be gracious to me, to rise up and show me compassion, but all too often I refuse to let You be my salvation. Instead of asking You for help, I rely on my own devices. Yet I am only blessed when I trust in You. Help me to trust You today and always. Amen.

Picture the scene in your mind: The Israelites are being pursued by the best of the Egyptian army, which is riding on swift horses and chariots, as the Israelites are walking on foot carrying their possessions. There are men, women and children, young and old in the crowd. Some are being carried because they are too weak or too feeble to proceed on their own. And as if the army behind them were not terrifying enough, there was a sea in front of them! There was literally no place for the Israelites to go!

Read Exodus 14:10-12. What did the people do as they saw Pharaoh approaching? What was their reaction? Explain what is happening as if you were an "on the scene" reporter covering this story for a national television news broadcast.

_____

_____

_____

_____

The people were terrified. They were questioning the Lord's love and mercy. They were wondering why they ever left Egypt. From a human standpoint, the situation looked hopeless. Yet Moses did not tell the Israelites to run or to surrender. He told them to *be still*. Read Moses' words in Exodus 14:13-14, and then continue your on-the-scene report of what is happening on the shore of the Red Sea.

_____

_____

_____

_____

Now read Exodus 14:15. What did the Lord say to Moses?

_____

_____

_____

_____

Moses told the people to be still. God told Moses to tell the Israelites to move on. What kind of stillness do you think Moses was talking about when he told the Israelites to "be still"?

_____

_____

_____

_____

Reading on in Exodus 14:16-18, what did God tell Moses to do, and what did God say He would do in return?

_____

_____

_____

_____

What does Exodus 14:17-18 tell us will happen to God's reputation as a result of what will happen in this situation?

_____

_____

_____

_____

How might God be using a difficult situation in your life—a situation that at the present moment seems impossible—to show His glory and might to those who don't believe in Him?

_____

_____

_____

_____

How can you be still before the Lord and also move forward in a present difficulty so that God's glory can shine through your circumstances?

_____

_____

_____

_____

What did you learn about stillness in today's lesson that you had not considered before?

_____

_____

_____

_____

_____

O Lord God, You call me to be still and know that You are God.
Yet stillness is difficult in the face of calamity. I will only be able to do
what You are asking me to do as You empower me. Amen.

SONGS OF PRAISE

Day
3

O Lord, You are my strength and my song; You are my salvation.
You are my God, and today I will exalt You and Your holy name. Amen.

Yesterday, you looked at the plight of the Israelites as they stood on the shore of the Red Sea. What appeared to be a certain calamity turned out to be a grand victory! When Moses reached out his staff, the waters parted and the Israelites walked across to the other side on dry land. When they were safely on the other side, we are told that Moses and the Israelites celebrated! Yet they were not celebrating victory because of their brave acts and mighty deeds.

Read Exodus 15:1-18 to discover who is getting all the praise and glory for this overwhelming success. As you read Moses' words, look for the word "still" as it applied to Israel's enemies (see v. 16). How is this still-ness different from being still before the Lord?

They were without power

_____

_____

Using Moses' wonderful song of praise as your template, compose your own song of praise to the Lord. Be sure to include the elements you see in Moses' song as he names the specific things God did for His people. How has God's unfailing love led you? How has He stretched out His mighty hand and defeated your foes—the things that stood between you and success in your journey?

_____

_____

_____

_____

_____

_____

_____

After writing your song of praise, turn to Exodus 6:6-8 and look at the promise God made to Moses before the Israelites left Egypt to begin their desert journey. How were God's actions on behalf of the Israelites as they stood by the banks of the Red Sea an affirmation of the promise contained in Exodus 6:6-8?

they could see what He had done

for them

_____

_____

How has God kept His word of promise to you as you have been faithful to keep Him first in all things? (You might want to consider the words of Matthew 6:33 as you answer this question.)

If we seek Him first all things

He will answer our prayers in His

time.

_____

_____

How has stillness been part of your keeping God first in all things?

We let Him be the Voice

O Lord, You are my refuge and my strength, a very present help in times of trouble. Thank You for Your Word and Your promises that allow me to be still and wait for You. Amen.

OUR REFUGE, OUR STRENGTH

Day 4

Lord God, I know that You are my rock and my fortress. Today I will be still and watch You do for me what I cannot do for myself. Amen.

This week's memory verse comes from Psalm 46, another beautiful song of praise to our God. Turn in your Bible to that psalm and prayerfully read its words, allowing God's majesty and power to fill your mind and soul. How does Psalm 46:1 describe God? Three specific attributes of God are given in this verse. As you look at these three attributes, think of a time when God has been all three of these things for you, and then write your reflections beside the attributes you listed.

refugia - strength - help

Attribute	Reflection

As a result of God being a fortress, a source of strength and an ever-present help, what will we not do, according to Psalm 46:2?

we will not fear

What specific examples are given in Psalm 46:2-3 that might give us reason to fear if God were not our fortress, our strength and our help?

the earth gives way
mountains fall in the sea
the waters roar & foam
the mountains quake

Whenever we see the little word "Selah" listed in the right margin of a verse in the Psalms, it is an invitation to stop and think about what was said in the portion of Scripture just read. How is stopping and thinking about what was said part of being still and knowing that God is God?

we must be still to think about
what we just read

The word "Selah" is used in Psalm 46 at the conclusion of verse 7. What are we being asked to ponder in this segment of the psalm?

know that God is with us and
He is our fortress & strength

Psalm 46:5 tells us that God is within her. What is being spoken of (referred to as "her") is the city of God. Drawing on what you have learned in earlier lessons, who is within us?

God

How has God kept you from falling during this session of First Place 4 Health? (Please explain your answer thoroughly. It will become part of your celebration story!)

I know if I fail sometimes God will help me pick up the pieces & get back on track

The invitation to stop and ponder what was just said is found again at the conclusion of Psalm 46:11. In many ways, this verse is the summary of the entire psalm. What one sentence could you use to summarize what God has done for you in First Place 4 Health? (This, too, can be part of your testimony.)

He has given me the spirit to continue my journey.

Lord God Almighty, because You are always with me, I can face each day with confidence. You are my Rock, my Refuge, my Strength and my Song; my ever-present help in time of trouble. Thank You for Your presence.

REMAIN IN GOD'S LOVE

*Most merciful Lord, today I give You all the thanks and praise for the good
things in my life. Without You, I can do no good thing. But in Your strength
and power, I can accomplish all the things You ask of me. Amen.*

Just before Jesus went to the cross, He spent time consoling His disciples.
Part of that consolation was the invitation to abide in Him. Turn to John
15 and read Jesus' words. Jesus begins His teaching with a statement
about who He is and who His Father is. What does John 15:1 tell us?

*I am the true vine and my Father
is the gardener*

Jesus declares that He is the vine. Why do you think Jesus uses this analogy to describe Himself? (In giving your answer, think about a vine in
relation to branches that have the potential of bearing fruit.)

*because He is being taught & pruned
by God the gardener*

Jesus goes on to say that His Father, the gardener, prunes the branches.
Why, according to John 15:2, is this pruning desirable?

*so that He may produce the
fruits of the Lord*

What hope can you take from the fact that God, the Master Gardener,
has taken the time to prune you?

He see's us all & teaches us

We need to be pruned in order to bear fruit for the Master. What else does John 15:4 tell us we must do in order to be fruitful servants?

We must remain in Him

How is continuing on in your journey after you have finished this session—and even after you have reached your goal weight—part of remaining in Jesus?

He will continue to teach us

John 15:7 tells us something specific that must happen if we are going to remain attached to Jesus, the vine. What are we told we must do?

We must remain in Him & His words remain in us.

Part of remaining in Jesus is allowing His words to remain in us. Scripture reading, Bible study and Scripture memorization are all part of this. How has being still before God as you have read and studied His Word helped you to celebrate success?

His words remain in us even in our failers

Jesus makes an awesome promise to us in John 15:7. What is that promise, and how does John 15:7 say the same thing as Matthew 6:33?

If we remain in Him, He will give us whatever we wish

John 15:8 tells us who will be the recipient of glory when we bear much fruit. Who will that be, and what can you do to give that person the glory for your success?

God
bear fruit & show ourselves to be
His Disciples

John 15:16 tells us that we did not choose Jesus, but rather He chose us to be His faithful, fruitful disciples. End today's lesson by thanking God that you have been chosen to be an instrument of God's love and grace.

> O Lord God, on my own I can do no good thing. All that I am and
> all that I have comes from You, my strength and my salvation!
> Today I will be still and remain in Your love. Amen.

Day 6 — REFLECTION AND APPLICATION

Gracious Lord, I know that You prune me so I can bear more fruit in Your kingdom. Thank You for giving me patient endurance to go through the process as You mold me into the image of Your Son, Jesus Christ. Amen.

During your studies this week, you have looked at the Lord's command to be still. Yet stillness is much, much more than a lack of physical activity! Being still before God is an act of the will, an intentional quieting of your heart and mind and soul, so that you can experience God's presence, hear His voice and remain steadfast in His love.

First Place 4 Health emphasizes the four-sided person. That's not to say that there are four separate compartments, each walled off from the other three, but rather that there are four different facets to the wonderfully made person God created in each of us. These four facets are part of the whole and complete person God fashioned us to be—and each facet is interrelated to the other three.

These four facets are listed below. Next to each one, write what stillness might look like in that area of your life and how stillness in that quadrant is connected to the stillness you are called to practice in the other three areas of your being.

Physical _____

_____

_____

_____

Mental _____

_____

_____

_____

Emotional _____

_____

_____

_____

Spiritual _____

_____

_____

_____

In which of these areas of your being is stillness the most problematic for you?

_____

_____

_____

_____

What can you do today to begin to be still before the Lord, even though you cannot go off to a deserted island and take a long rest?

_____

_____

_____

_____

How does the fact that God's Holy Spirit dwells in you give you assurance and quiet your troubled spirit?

_____

_____

_____

_____

> *Gracious God, You call me to be still. I know that unless I am willing to listen to Your voice and obey Your will, I will continue to rely on my own strength and power. Today, O Lord, I will put my trust in You. Amen.*

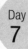

REFLECTION AND APPLICATION

Merciful and loving Lord, today I will rest secure in Your love and meditate on Your Word. You are indeed a God who is faithful! Amen.

At the beginning of this study, you were asked to list one way in which you wished to experience God at a deeper level—to know Him more intimately in that way. Review how you asked God to reveal Himself to you during your *Celebrate Success* journey. Now think back over the past 10 weeks. How has God been faithful to show Himself to you? (Some ways will be obvious; others will be subtle changes you could easily miss unless you give this exercise careful thought.)

_____

_____

_____

_____

_____

_____

_____

_____

After you have completed your reflection, end your quiet time by thanking the God of heaven and earth for revealing Himself to you in new and exciting ways as you have studied His Word and lived in His grace.

> *O Lord, if I had to depend on myself, I would be lost. But You assure me that You are my strength; therefore, I can be weak and vulnerable before You. You are the one who gives me what I need so that I can celebrate success in all areas of my life. You are the one who deserves to be exalted. Amen.*

Group Prayer Requests

first place
4health

Today's Date: _____

Name	Request
Shelly Long	
Eugene Mann	
Tami's Dad	
Lee King - recovery	
Jone Icenbice	
Karen —	hives

Results

_____

_____

_____

_____

_____

_____

time to celebrate!

To help shape your brief victory celebration testimony, work through the following questions in your prayer journal:

Day One: List some of the benefits you have gained by allowing the Lord to transform your life through this 12-week First Place 4 Health session. Be sure to list benefits you have received in the physical, mental, emotional and spiritual realms of your being.

Day Two: In what ways have you most significantly changed *mentally*? Have you seen a shift in the ways you think about yourself, food, your relationships or God? How has Scripture memory been a part of these shifts?

Day Three: In what ways have you most significantly changed *emotionally*? Have you begun to identify how your feelings influence your relationship to food and exercise? What are you doing to stay aware of your emotions, both positive and negative?

Day Four: In what ways have you most significantly changed *spiritually*? How has your relationship with God deepened? How has drawing closer to Him made a difference in the other three areas of your life?

Day Five: In what ways have you most significantly changed *physically*? Have you met or exceeded your weight/measurement goals? How has your health improved the past 12 weeks?

Day Six: Was there one person in your First Place 4 Health group who was particularly encouraging to you? How did their kindness make a difference in your First Place 4 Health journey?

Day Seven: Summarize the previous six questions into a one-page testimony, or "faith story," to share at your group's victory celebration.

May our gracious Lord bless and keep you as you continue to keep Him first in all things!

Celebrate Success
leader discussion guide

For in-depth information, guidance and helpful tips about leading a successful First Place 4 Health group, study the *First Place 4 Health Leader's Guide*. In it, you will find valuable answers to most of your questions, as well as personal insights from many First Place 4 Health group leaders.

For the group meetings in this session, be sure to read and consider each week's discussion topics several days before the meeting—some questions and activities require supplies and/or planning to complete. Also, if you are leading a large group, plan to break into smaller groups for discussion and then come together as a large group to share your answers and responses. Choose a capable leader for each small group who can keep discussions focused and on track (and be sure each group records its answers!).

week one: welcome to *Celebrate Success*

During this first week, welcome the members to your group, provide a brief overview of the First Place 4 Health program, explain what is expected of the participants at each of the weekly meetings and collect the Member Surveys. (See the *First Place 4 Health Leader's Guide* for a detailed outline of how to conduct the first week's meeting.)

week two: celebrate love and faithfulness

Begin today's session by asking the participants in your group to describe the images the words "celebrate success" bring to their hearts and minds. Be sure to give each person in your group an opportunity to talk rather than letting one or two monopolize the conversation.

Next, go around the room and ask your group what images and visions the words "well done, good and faithful servant" brought up for them. Once again, give everyone an opportunity to talk.

Talk to your group about why Jesus spoke in parables and what those parables were designed to do. Remember, some in your group may be new to Jesus' teaching stories.

Ask your group to describe how First Place 4 Health might be part of their calling to serve God with the talents they have been given.

It is very important that your group understand the truth of 1 Corinthians 3:16 and 1 Corinthians 6:19-20. Be sure to allow plenty of time to talk about the Temple of the Holy Spirit.

There may be those in your group who are confused about "judgment" versus "accountability." Be sure that you understand the difference between these two terms so that you can answer questions appropriately.

Have someone in your group read Psalm 139, verses 1-4 and 13-16, and then lead a discussion about how each of us are "fearfully and wonderfully made."

God has given us all that we need to be faithful and fruitful servants! During the Day Four study, participants were asked to read verses that describe aspects of God's faithfulness and then talk about how that aspect of God's love and faithfulness allows them to be faithful stewards. Spend some time reviewing this exercise with your group.

Knowing God, as He reveals Himself in the pages of Scripture, is the most important work we will ever do as Christians. Talk to your group about the importance of knowing God—and how they can learn about who God is in the pages of the Bible.

End today's lesson by reading Ephesians 3:14-21 as your prayer for the group during this session of First Place 4 Health.

week three: celebrate hope for a better tomorrow

On Day One, participants read how Jesus told His disciples about the importance of considering the cost. On a whiteboard or newspaper flip chart, write the words "consider the cost" and then lead a group discussion about the "hidden" costs of participation in First Place 4 Health. Don't get focused on material costs, because they are minor when compared to the time and energy it takes to be faithful to the First Place 4 Health program.

On Day Two, the group studied Moses and the tent of meeting. This lesson has foundational principles that help to establish a quiet time with God. Begin the discussion by having someone in the group read Exodus 33:7-11. Ask your group to talk about what they are doing to pitch a "tent of meeting" and why it is important that the tent be a distance away from "the camp" where they live and work.

Many are uncomfortable with the idea of being open about their quiet time with God. Ask your group how allowing others to know about the importance of their relationship with God is a hidden cost of being in First Place 4 Health.

When Moses went inside the tent, the cloud covered the entrance. It is awesome to realize that God values quiet time with us! Ask your group to talk about this awesome reality and what that fact means to them.

Jeremiah 9:23 lists three things the world boasts about. List those three things on your whiteboard or flip chart and ask your group to give you examples of all three.

Talk about the cost involved in the three things the world values (from your previous question). The group will find that none of these things are "instant" accomplishments!

Your group has drawn sketches of their "tent of meeting." Give everyone an opportunity to share what their meeting place looks like and what they have inside their tent.

On Day Seven, your group listed how the four aspects of God's love, from this week's memory verse, are applicable to First Place 4 Health. Review this exercise with your group.

week four: celebrate our weakness

It is difficult to accept that we are flawed human beings until we realize that the flaws are what allow God's grace to flow through us. Begin your study this week by talking about how the world would like us to consider that our greatest strength is having no weaknesses.

Ask someone in your group to read 2 Corinthians 4:7. Lead a discussion about being jars of clay.

In 2 Corinthians 12:7-10, Paul talks about his "thorn in the flesh." Put the words "painful," "powerful" and "persistent" on your whiteboard or flip chart and talk about how these same three words can apply to the malady called "compulsive overeating."

Many people don't like to admit to being compulsive overeaters, even though they are carrying the effects of that malady around with them. Talk about how compulsive overeating affects us physically, mentally, emotionally and spiritually.

Just as parables may be new to some in your group, the concept of paradox may be new as well. Spend some time explaining paradox (if you are unsure about how to do that, talk to your pastor or a seasoned Bible teacher before you try to explain it to your group).

Ask someone in your group, someone with the gift of reading Scripture, to read Mary's beautiful Magnificat. Afterwards, lead a discussion about what Mary is saying—and why.

Go over the chart of paradoxes in the Day Four study, being sure that everyone has correctly understood those statements.

We all fall into the "perfection" trap from time to time. Talk to your group about the difference between "excellence" and "perfection."

During the Day Six reflection, participants looked at the four types of people whom Jesus came to rescue from a life of shame and disgrace. Talk about these four types of people, and then ask your group to talk about how they identified—or didn't identify—with them.

week five: celebrate unity

When we speak of unity, most of us think of groups who are of "one mind." Begin your group by talking about the things you have in common as a group.

Ask the group to share their answers on what impressed them most about the story of the heroic four friends. Ask if they can recall a time when someone "carried" them to Jesus.

On Day Two, participants looked at Hebrews 4:12. Ask members if they can recite a Scripture that has brought healing or comfort to them in a time of need. The Scriptures tell us that God's Word is living and active.

On Day Three, participants read Isaiah 58:6-12. Ask the group to share some of the things God would do if they were obedient to minister to others. Ask them to share from the list what is most precious to them.

On Day Six, participants looked at the truth of Romans 8:1. Have each person in your group repeat that verse out loud.

During the Day Seven reflection, participants were asked to make a collage that depicted the virtue they would like to put on. Allow enough time for the group members to share the pictures they collected.

End your session on a note of hope. Jesus Christ has saved us from this war. He has saved us from this body of death!

week six: celebrate patience and preparation

Read Psalm 40:1 and talk about the sequence that led to God hearing David's voice.

Ask someone in your group to read Psalm 34:18, and then talk about where the Lord is when we are brokenhearted.

On Day Two, the study talked about patience as it applies to prayer. Be sure your group grasps this concept, because patience with the process is essential to success in First Place 4 Health!

Philippians 1:6 is a wonderful message of hope. Ask your group what those words mean to their First Place 4 Health efforts.

Esther is a vivid example of the preparation we need to engage in as we seek the king's favor. Be sure to tie in Esther's one year of preparation with the year-long commitment that members are asked to make in First Place 4 Health.

The Week Six memory verse is about portion. Although we usually think of portion in terms of food, with God as our portion, what He gives us is always enough. Ask your group how that truth relates to the Live-It plan.

On your whiteboard or flip chart, list the elements of the First Place 4 Health acrostic that explains how we pray (F.I.R.S.T.). Talk about how all those elements are found in Daniel's prayer.

Many of us question what God is using us for in His kingdom. The Day Seven reflection gives some tools for figuring out how we can discern God's will. Review this exercise with your group.

week seven: celebrate God's dwelling place

The word "defile" is not a word we use much these days. Come to your group prepared to talk about what "defile" means as it relates to our relationship with God.

The Book of Haggai has great application for those who are participating in First Place 4 Health. However, those who want to take a more "literal" interpretation of the Bible may have difficulty with this concept. It is important to explain that the book of Haggai was about an actual Temple that was lying in ruins, but that we can apply it to our bodies by way of analogy.

Procrastination is what stands between most of us and First Place 4 Health success. We know what to do, but somehow we don't get around to doing it. Talk about how procrastination threatens First Place 4 Health success.

On Day Two, participants looked at the five ways in which God speaks to us. Write these five ways on your whiteboard or flip chart. Have your group discuss how God uses First Place 4 Health to speak to them in those ways.

Haggai talks about never having "enough." Look at the things God tells us we will never have enough of until we honor Him. Talk with your group about how these things are representative of our addictive society.

When we come to the realization that we are destroying God's Temple with food, our first reaction is often denial. Talk to your group about this fact and any way in which they might be resisting the truth presented in God's Word.

Most of us don't like the idea of hard work when it comes to repairing the Lord's temple, our bodies. Ask your group what kind of hard work they may need to do to bring God's temple back into good repair.

In order to succeed, there are always things we must give up. This, too, is part of the cost of obedient discipleship. Have your group talk about what they will need to give up in order to succeed in First Place 4 Health.

Be sure each person in your group signed and dated the covenant contained in the Day Seven reflection.

week eight: celebrate with singing

When we think of encouragement, we usually think of words said to others, but as our study this week revealed, we also encourage others by the way we treat them. As you lead today's meeting, think about how the group members represent a wide spectrum of spiritual levels, and do everything you can to speak to all in an uplifting and inspiring way.

Because of who we are in Christ, we have so much to be thankful for and sing about. Ask your class to share some of the treasures Christ has left for them from the introduction to Day One.

Ask the members of your group to share what the word "hope" means to them from the exercise on Day One.

No doubt all group members have experienced or are presently experiencing some degree of suffering. Lead a discussion from their findings from Romans 8:18.

Ask your class to discuss what they discovered about the relationship between glory and suffering and how God is the silent partner in every conversation.

Have a member of your group read 1 Corinthians 13:4-7, and then lead a discussion about what the people in the group learned from studying the apostle Paul's words this week.

Your group was asked to reflect on how faith, hope and love are part of success in First Place 4 Health. Invite them to share their thoughts with the group.

week nine: celebrate God's goodness

Begin your meeting by having the group recite Philippians 4:4-7 in unison. You might want to make photocopies of the verse so that everyone can read from the same translation.

Talk about Paul's circumstances when he wrote those verses. A Bible dictionary can help you research the topic.

Lead a discussion about how rejoicing in the Lord is different from rejoicing in our circumstances.

The reason for our hope is that God is always present with us. Talk to your group about that precious truth.

Anxiety can have bad effects on our ability to control our eating, be diligent with exercise, and spend quality time with God each day. Talk with your group about how anxiety is the opposite of joy.

Prayer is always the answer! Go through the elements Paul says are to be part of our prayers. Ask the group how they can apply these truths to their First Place 4 Health disciplines.

Write "my understanding" on your whiteboard or flip chart. Ask how these two words keep us from trusting God.

Day Five talks about the things we are to "think on." Go over this list with your group as it relates to First Place 4 Health.

Review the invitation listed for the Day Seven Reflection. Ask each person to identify which invitation they will accept and what they are willing to do to say yes to God's goodness and love.

week ten: celebrate worship

We are saved from the bondage of sin so that we can worship God! Lead a discussion about how we worship God in our everyday lives.

Although we think of "festival" and "celebration" as two different things, the Bible uses the words interchangeably. Talk to your group about the meaning of both words.

Ask your group members to tell about a time when they argued with their Maker as it related to caring for themselves.

Ask someone in your group to read Psalm 23 and then talk about the Lord as Shepherd.

Excess is part of the society we live in; however, excess is an affront to God. Talk about the various forms of excess—and how God views it.

Talk about excess in the four quadrants of life. Some may struggle with spiritual excess answers. Spiritual excess is taking in more each day than we can digest and assimilate. Often, this is a cover-up for rebellion.

On Day Seven, each group member was asked to do a "whole body prayer." Ask your group to describe that experience.

End your session by having the group read Psalm 95:6 in unison. As before, provide everyone the same translation to read.

week eleven: celebrate stillness

During the Day One lessons, the group was asked to read Exodus 14:10-18 and give reports on what was happening by the shore of the Red Sea as if they were on-the-scene reporters. Have the group members read these accounts—dramatically—to the group.

Ask your group to share whether or not they could have been calm, given the circumstances—and have them explain why or why not!

Moses' song in Exodus 15:1-18 is a wonderful account of God's deliverance of the Israelites from bondage. Ask someone in your group to read this passage to the group.

Ask each person in the group to talk about the passage in Moses' song that was especially meaningful for them.

Psalm 46:1 lists three attributes that David uses to describe God. Write each of these attributes on a whiteboard or flip chart, and then talk about what each attribute means, especially as it applies to First Place 4 Health participation.

The description of remaining in God's love is a wonderful opportunity to discuss future plans for your First Place 4 Health group. Begin that discussion now.

Talk about how all four aspects of our being can be "still before the Lord" and how one quadrant affects the other three.

End your group session with a time of stillness. Have the group use the words of this week's memory verse to engage in a mini-Lectio Divina.

week twelve: time to celebrate!

Even though most of your meeting this week will be a victory celebration, take some time at the beginning of the meeting to talk about how much God loves each person in the group and how they are called to love their brothers and sisters in Christ. (See "Planning a Victory Celebration" in the *First Place 4 Health Leader's Guide* for ideas about throwing a successful celebration for your group.)

For the rest of the study time, allow each member to tell his or her *Celebrate Success* story. Give members an equal opportunity to share the goals they set for themselves at the beginning of the session and talk about the challenges and good things God has done for them throughout the process. Don't allow anyone to monopolize the time; the quiet members need an opportunity to share their stories and successes. Even those who have not met their goals have still been part of the journey, so allow them to share and talk about why they did not succeed.

Making a commitment to continue in First Place 4 Health is an important part of victory. Be sure to talk about your group's future plans, and make each person feel welcome to continue the journey with you.

End your victory celebration by reading aloud Paul's prayer for the Ephesians found in Ephesians 3:14-21, a wonderful benediction. Make Paul's words your prayer for your group as they conclude *Celebrate Success*!

First Place 4 Health menu plans

Each menu plan is based on approximately 1,400 to 1,500 calories per day. All recipe and menu exchanges were determined using the Master-Cook software, a program that accesses a database containing more than 6,000 food items prepared using the United States Department of Agriculture (USDA) publications and information from food manufacturers. As with any nutritional program, MasterCook calculates the nutritional values of the recipes based on ingredients. Nutrition may vary due to how the food is prepared, where the food comes from, soil content, season, ripeness, processing and method of preparation. For these reasons, please use the recipes and menu plans as approximate guides. Consult a physician and/or a registered dietitian before starting a weight-loss program.

For those who need more calories, add the following to the 1,400-calorie plan:

- 1,800 calories: 2 ounce equivalent of meat, 3 ounce equivalent of bread, $^1/_2$ cup vegetable serving, 1 tsp. fat

- 2,000 calories: 2 ounce equivalent of meat, 4 ounce equivalent of bread, $^1/_2$ cup vegetable serving, 3 tsp. fat

- 2,200 calories: 2 ounce equivalent of meat, 5 ounce equivalent of bread, $^1/_2$ cup vegetable serving, $^1/_2$ cup fruit serving, 5 tsp. fat

- 2,400 calories: 2 ounce equivalent of meat, 6 ounce equivalent of bread, 1 cup vegetable serving, $^1/_2$ cup fruit serving, 6 tsp. fat

First Week Grocery List

Produce
- ❑ alfalfa sprouts
- ❑ apples
- ❑ bananas
- ❑ blackberries
- ❑ broccoli
- ❑ cantaloupe
- ❑ carrots
- ❑ cauliflower
- ❑ celery
- ❑ cherry tomatoes
- ❑ cilantro
- ❑ cucumbers
- ❑ garlic cloves
- ❑ green beans
- ❑ green bell peppers
- ❑ iceberg lettuce
- ❑ lime
- ❑ mango
- ❑ mushrooms
- ❑ orange
- ❑ parsley, fresh
- ❑ peaches
- ❑ pear
- ❑ pineapple
- ❑ plums
- ❑ potatoes
- ❑ raspberries
- ❑ red bell peppers
- ❑ red onions
- ❑ romaine lettuce
- ❑ spinach
- ❑ squash
- ❑ scallions
- ❑ tomatoes
- ❑ zucchini

Baking Products
- ❑ all-fruit spread
- ❑ apple cider
- ❑ applesauce, unsweetened
- ❑ barbeque sauce
- ❑ basil, fresh
- ❑ black pepper, freshly ground
- ❑ cayenne pepper
- ❑ cayenne pepper sauce
- ❑ chili powder
- ❑ cooking sherry
- ❑ croutons
- ❑ cumin
- ❑ Dijon mustard
- ❑ dill, dried
- ❑ flour
- ❑ Italian salad dressing, light
- ❑ lemon juice
- ❑ lime juice
- ❑ olive oil
- ❑ olives
- ❑ oregano
- ❑ raisins
- ❑ ranch salad dressing, reduced-fat
- ❑ red kidney beans
- ❑ salsa
- ❑ salt
- ❑ strawberry jam
- ❑ sun-dried tomatoes
- ❑ taco seasoning

❑ Thousand Island salad
dressing, reduced-fat
❑ thyme, dried
❑ tomato juice
❑ vinegar

Breads and Cereals
❑ bagels
❑ breadsticks
❑ cornbread
❑ crackers
❑ dinner rolls, whole-wheat
❑ egg noodles
❑ English muffins
❑ flour tortillas, lowfat
❑ fortified cold cereal
❑ Grape-Nuts® cereal
❑ instant oatmeal, flavored
❑ oat muffin, reduced-fat
❑ rice cakes
❑ Rice Chex® cereal
❑ rice pilaf
❑ rye bread
❑ shell macaroni
❑ tortilla chips, nonfat
❑ walnuts

Canned Foods
❑ 17-oz. cannellini beans (1 can)
❑ chicken broth, low-sodium
(1 can)
❑ 4-oz. water-packed tuna
(2 cans)

Dairy Products
❑ Colby Jack cheese, lowfat
❑ cottage cheese, 2-percent
❑ eggs
❑ margarine, reduced-calorie
❑ mayonnaise, reduced-calorie
❑ milk, nonfat
❑ pepper Jack cheese
❑ raspberry-apple juice
❑ sour cream, light
❑ yogurt, nonfat

Frozen Foods
❑ broccoli
❑ frozen yogurt, nonfat no-
sugar-added chocolate
❑ Lean Cuisine Pasta Alfredo®
❑ waffles, frozen

Seafood and Meat
❑ (8) chicken breasts, boneless
with skin (4 oz. each)
❑ flounder (3 oz.)
❑ ground beef, lean (1 lb.)
❑ pork loin, lean boneless
(2 lbs.)
❑ (2) sirloin steaks, lean 1/2-
inch thick (6 oz. each)
❑ turkey breast, skinless,
boneless (2 oz.)
❑ turkey meat, light
❑ (4) veal chops, lean, center-
cut (1 1/4 to 1 1/2 lbs. each)

First Week Meals and Recipes

DAY 1

Breakfast

2 lowfat frozen waffles
$^1/_2$ cup unsweetened applesauce
  (to top waffle)
2 tbsp. raisins

1 pkg. Equal® (if desired, to
  sweeten applesauce)
1 cup nonfat milk

Nutritional Information: 372 calories; 6g fat (14.3% calories from fat); 13g protein; 68g carbohydrate; 4g dietary fiber; 27mg cholesterol; 658mg sodium.

Lunch

Turkey Salad

2 oz. skinless, boneless cooked
  turkey breast, diced
$^1/_4$ cup chopped celery
2 tbsp. chopped red onion

2 tsp. chopped spinach leaves
1 tsp. fresh lemon juice
2 tsp. reduced-calorie mayonnaise

Serve with:

$^1/_2$ cup tomato slices
$^1/_2$ cup cucumber slices
2 tsp. light Italian salad dressing

2 rice cakes
1 pear

Combine ingredients. Serves 1.

Nutritional Information: 303 calories; 5g fat (14.8% calories from fat); 17g protein; 51g carbohydrate; 7g dietary fiber; 37mg cholesterol; 260mg sodium.

Dinner

Steak Tacos

1 lime
1 tbsp. taco seasoning
(2) 6-oz. $^1/_2$-inch-thick lean
  sirloin steaks
$^1/_2$ cup lowfat Colby Jack
  cheese, shredded

light sour cream
(8) 6-inch lowfat flour tortillas
shredded lettuce
1 cup prepared salsa

Serve with:

3/4 cup grilled fresh pineapple wedges or canned spears

1 cup sliced cucumbers marinated in light Italian dressing per person

Squeeze lime juice over all surfaces of meat. Sprinkle each side of meat with taco seasoning. Place steaks on a grill over a medium-hot fire or under broiler. Grill or broil to desired doneness (4 minutes each side for medium). While steaks are cooking, warm tortillas and salsa. Divide cheese evenly on top of steaks. Cut each steak into 8 pieces. Serve 2 pieces of steak with a tortilla and salsa. Garnish with shredded lettuce and light sour cream. Serves 4.

Nutritional Information: 615 calories; 19g fat (27.5% calories from fat); 30g protein; 84g carbohydrate; 8g dietary fiber; 58mg cholesterol; 1,214mg sodium.

DAY 2

Breakfast

1 pkg. instant flavored oatmeal with 4 walnut halves, chopped

1/2 banana
1 cup nonfat milk

Nutritional Information: 439 calories; 6g fat (11.4% calories from fat); 22g protein; 78g carbohydrate; 10g dietary fiber; 4mg cholesterol; 945mg sodium.

Lunch

Broiled Flounder
3 oz. flounder, broiled

Serve with:

3/4 cup boiled new potatoes with 1 tsp. reduced-calorie margarine and minced fresh parsley
1 cup steamed zucchini slices
1 iceberg lettuce wedge

1 tbsp. reduced-fat Thousand Island salad dressing
(1) 1-oz. breadstick
small orange

Nutritional Information: 401 calories; 7g fat (14.6% calories from fat); 25g protein; 62g carbohydrate; 7g dietary fiber; 42mg cholesterol; 368mg sodium.

Dinner

Chicken Breast with Raspberry Sauce

2 tsp. olive oil
1 red onion, thinly sliced
(4) 4-oz. boneless chicken
  breasts with skin
$1/2$ tsp. salt

$2^1/_2$ cups fresh or 1 cup
  frozen raspberries
$1/_4$ tsp. freshly ground
  black pepper
1 cup raspberry-apple juice

Serve with:

$2/_3$ cup cooked rice pilaf

1 cup steamed broccoli with
  1 tsp. melted margarine

Heat oil in a large nonstick skillet. Add onion and sauté 2 minutes; do not brown. Remove onion and set aside. Season the flesh side of breast with salt and pepper; add to pan and cook over medium heat only until each side is lightly browned. Add juice to pan and continue cooking until chicken is cooked through, about 12 minutes. Remove chicken from pan. Add onions to skillet; cook until liquid has a syrupy consistency. Add raspberries and heat through. Remove skin from chicken before serving and serve breast topped with sauce. Serves 2.

Nutritional Information: 453 calories; 7g fat (14.6% calories from fat); 36g protein; 62g carbohydrate; 11g dietary fiber; 66mg cholesterol; 436mg sodium.

DAY 3

Breakfast

1 medium reduced-fat oat muffin
1 medium fresh peach or other fruit

1 cup nonfat artificially
  sweetened fruit-flavored yogurt

Nutritional Information: 326 calories; 7g fat (18.8% calories from fat); 15g protein; 53g carbohydrate; 5g dietary fiber; 25mg cholesterol; 398mg sodium.

Lunch

Broccoli Bisque with Egg Salad Muffin

2 cups frozen chopped broccoli
$1/_2$ cup low-sodium chicken broth

$1/_2$ cup nonfat milk
2 boiled egg whites

1 boiled whole egg, chopped
1 tbsp. finely chopped celery

2 tsp. reduced-calorie mayonnaise
English muffin, toasted

Serve with: 1 small apple

In a small bowl, combine boiled egg whites, boiled whole egg, celery and mayonnaise. Scoop onto a toasted English muffin. Combine broccoli, broth and milk in food processor and puree until smooth. Transfer to medium saucepan and cook until heated. Season with salt and pepper if desired. Serves 1.

Nutritional Information: 493 calories; 11g fat (18.9% calories from fat); 38g protein; 72g carbohydrate; 15g dietary fiber; 218mg cholesterol; 655mg sodium.

....

Dinner

Mustard Chicken
(4) 4-oz. boneless chicken breasts
$1/2$ tsp. dried dill
$1/2$ tsp. salt
$1/4$ tsp. black pepper
$1/2$ cup apple cider

2 tbsp. Dijon mustard
1 tbsp. olive oil
2 cloves garlic, minced
$1/3$ cup fresh parsley, chopped
$1/4$ cup water

Serve with:
$1/2$ cup garlic mashed potatoes
1 cup sautéed squash with pepper

1 breadstick per person

Preheat oven to 350°F. On a cutting board, cover each breast with plastic wrap and pound with a meat mallet until the breast is $1/2$-inch thick. Heat oil in a large nonstick skillet; add garlic and cook for 2 minutes over medium heat. Add chicken breasts and brown for 3 minutes on each side. Transfer chicken to a $11/2$-quart casserole dish. Put cider, water, mustard, dill, salt and pepper into the skillet, and then stir to mix with the chicken drippings. Bring to a boil and cook for 1 minute. Pour over chicken in casserole dish. Cover and bake 20 minutes. Add parsley, baste with sauce, and bake an additional 5 minutes. Serves 4.

Nutritional Information: 370 calories; 10g fat (23.8% calories from fat); 33g protein; 38g carbohydrate; 5g dietary fiber; 68mg cholesterol; 834mg sodium.

DAY 4

Breakfast

$^3/_4$ cup Rice Chex® cereal
1 cup nonfat milk
$^1/_2$ banana

$^1/_2$ English muffin
$^1/_2$ tsp. reduced-calorie margarine
1 tsp. all-fruit spread

Nutritional Information: 293 calories; 2g fat (5.4% calories from fat); 14g protein; 57g carbohydrate; 4g dietary fiber; 4mg cholesterol; 491mg sodium.

Lunch

Tuna Salad Nicoise
2 cups shredded romaine lettuce
1 tomato, quartered
$^1/_2$ cup cooked green beans

4 oz. water-packed tuna
4 large pitted olives
light Italian salad dressing

Serve with:
2 long breadsticks

1 banana

In a medium bowl, combine lettuce leaves, tomato, green beans, drained tuna, olives and 1 tablespoon light Italian salad dressing. Serves 1.

Nutritional Information: 393 calories; 7g fat (16.3% calories from fat); 36g protein; 50g carbohydrate; 9g dietary fiber; 34mg cholesterol; 755mg sodium.

Dinner

Crockpot Cider Pork Stew
2 lbs. lean boneless pork loin
1 tsp. salt
3 tbsp. flour
$^1/_4$ tsp. dried thyme
$^1/_4$ tsp. pepper
3 cups carrots, sliced
2 large onions, cubed

2 cups apple cider
$^1/_2$ cup cold water
3 cups potatoes, cubed
2 apples, cubed
1 tbsp. vinegar
$^1/_4$ cup flour

Serve with:
2-inch square of cornbread
1 cup steamed broccoli

1 cup steamed cauliflower

Cut pork into cubes. Combine the 3 tablespoons of flour, salt, thyme and pepper and toss with the meat. Put the carrots, potatoes, onions and apples in a crockpot. Top with meat cubes. Combine the apple cider and vinegar and pour over the meat. Cover and cook on low for 8 to 10 hours. Turn the crockpot to high. Combine $1/4$ cup flour and $1/2$ cup cold water and blend well. Stir into the liquid in the crockpot, and then cover and cook for 15 to 20 minutes or until thickened. Season to taste. Serves 8.

Nutritional Information: 531 calories; 13g fat (21.3% calories from fat); 35g protein; 71g carbohydrate; 9g dietary fiber; 99mg cholesterol; 814mg sodium.

DAY 5

Breakfast

$1/3$ medium cantaloupe
  or honeydew melon
1 cup nonfat artificially sweetened
  pineapple-flavored yogurt
  (to top melon)

$1/4$ cup Grape-Nuts® cereal
  (sprinkled on yogurt)

Nutritional Information: 281 calories; 1g fat (3.7% calories from fat); 15g protein; 57g carbohydrate; 5g dietary fiber; 3mg cholesterol; 345mg sodium.

Lunch

Bean and Salsa Salad
$1/2$ cup cooked red kidney beans
$1^1/2$ oz. shredded pepper
  Jack cheese
$1/2$ cup finely chopped red onion
$1/4$ cup salsa

1 tsp. fresh lime juice
spinach leaves
2 tbsp. light sour cream
1 tsp. minced fresh cilantro

Serve with:
1 oz. nonfat tortilla chips

$1/2$ small mango

In a small bowl, combine red kidney beans, shredded pepper Jack cheese, red onion, salsa and fresh lime juice. Line plate with spinach leaves and top with bean mixture, light sour cream and cilantro. Serves 1.

Nutritional Information: 613 calories; 16g fat (23.0% calories from fat); 34g protein; 88g carbohydrate; 19g dietary fiber; 47mg cholesterol; 576mg sodium.

Dinner

Seared Veal Chops with Sun-dried Tomatoes

(4) $1^1/_4$-lb. to $1^1/_2$-lb.
  lean center-cut veal chops
$^1/_4$ cup sun-dried tomatoes
1 cup tomato juice
$^1/_2$ cup water

2 tbsp. fresh basil, chopped
  (or 1 tsp. dried leaf basil)
$^1/_2$ tsp. cayenne pepper sauce
salt and pepper to taste

Serve with:

$^1/_2$ cup Lean Cuisine Pasta Alfredo®
$^1/_2$ cup mixed vegetables

1 whole-wheat dinner roll

Trim and discard excess fat from chops. Sear the chops in a frying pan. When the chops are browned, add the juice, water, cayenne pepper sauce, salt and pepper. Cover tightly and simmer for 15 minutes. Add the sun-dried tomatoes and cook for 10 minutes. Add basil and continue to cook for 8 minutes. Add remaining basil and cook for 3 more minutes. Spoon some of the tomatoes and basil over the veal to serve. Serves 4.

Nutritional Information: 472 calories; 17g fat (32.1% calories from fat); 34g protein; 47g carbohydrate; 8g dietary fiber; 119mg cholesterol; 1,114mg sodium.

DAY 6

Breakfast

1 cup fortified cold cereal
$^1/_2$ small mango

1 cup nonfat milk

Nutritional Information: 260 calories; 1g fat (4% calories from fat); 12g protein; 54g carbohydrate; 5g dietary fiber; 4mg cholesterol; 131mg sodium.

Lunch

Cottage Cheese Lunch

$^1/_2$ cup 2-percent cottage cheese
$^1/_4$ cup alfalfa sprouts

$^1/_2$ tbsp. chopped scallions

Serve with:

4-oz. no-sugar-added chocolate
  nonfat frozen yogurt

2 slices rye bread, toasted with
  2 tsp. reduced-calorie margarine

$^1/_2$ cup each red and green bell pepper strips with 2 tbsp. reduced-fat ranch dressing

2 plums

Combine all. Serves 1.

Nutritional Information: 439 calories; 12g fat (24.3% calories from fat); 24g protein; 61g carbohydrate; 8g dietary fiber; 11mg cholesterol; 1,217mg sodium.

....

Dinner

Beef and Noodles in BBQ Sauce
4 oz. egg noodles
2 tbsp. reduced-calorie margarine
$^3/_4$ cup onions, diced
1 lb. lean ground beef
1 lb. mushrooms, sliced

$^3/_4$ cup water
2 egg yolks
3 tbsp. BBQ sauce
2 tbsp. cooking sherry

Serve with: spinach salad topped with croutons and a light salad dressing

Put the noodles into a heat-resistant mixing bowl and cover with boiling water. Set aside for 20 minutes and then drain. In a frying pan, melt the margarine, add the onions and sauté for 5 minutes or so. Add the beef, mushrooms and noodles. Increase the heat to high and cook for another 5 minutes, stirring constantly. Add the water and cook another 10 minutes over low heat. In a small bowl, mix together the egg yolks, BBQ sauce and sherry. Scoop a few spoonfuls of the meat mixture into the bowl containing the egg mixture. Turn the contents of the bowl into the skillet. Heat gently while stirring. Serve over the noodles. Serves 4.

Nutritional Information: 564 calories; 31g fat (50.7% calories from fat); 31g protein; 38g carbohydrate; 5g dietary fiber; 218mg cholesterol; 358mg sodium.

DAY 7

....

Breakfast
1 small (2-oz.) bagel
1 tsp. strawberry jam
$^3/_4$ cup blackberries (mix into yogurt)

1 cup artificially sweetened, mixed berry nonfat yogurt

Nutritional Information: 343 calories; 2g fat (4.4% calories from fat); 17g protein; 67g carbohydrate; 8g dietary fiber; 3mg cholesterol; 437mg sodium.

Lunch

Tuna-pasta Salad

$^1/_2$ cup cooked shell macaroni
4 oz. water-packed tuna
6 cherry tomatoes, halved

$^1/_4$ cup diced red onion
1 tbsp. light Italian salad dressing

Serve with:

$^1/_2$ cup each carrots and celery sticks
1 medium peach

2 oz. whole-wheat roll with 1 tsp.
  reduced-calorie margarine

Combine all ingredients in a medium bowl. Serves 1.

Nutritional Information: 426 calories; 7g fat (13.7% calories from fat); 37g protein; 56g carbohydrate; 8g dietary fiber; 35mg cholesterol; 746mg sodium.

Dinner

White Turkey Chili

$1^1/_2$ cups onion, chopped
$^1/_2$ cup green bell pepper, chopped
2 cloves garlic, minced
$^1/_2$ tsp. olive oil
1 tsp. cumin
(1) 17-oz. can of cannellini beans,
  drained and rinsed

2 cups turkey light meat, cooked
  and cubed
1 tsp. chili powder
$^1/_4$ tsp. cayenne pepper
$^1/_4$ tsp. salt
1 cup chicken broth
1 tsp. oregano

Serve with:

8 crackers

green salad

In a 3-quart saucepan, cook the onions, bell peppers and garlic in oil over medium heat until tender. Add cumin, oregano, chili powder, cayenne pepper and salt. Cook for 1 minute. Stir in beans and turkey. Bring to a boil, reduce heat and simmer uncovered for 30 minutes or until slightly thickened. Serves 8.

Nutritional Information: 438 calories; 7g fat (14.3% calories from fat); 31g protein; 65g carbohydrate; 15g dietary fiber; 26mg cholesterol; 511mg sodium.

Second Week Grocery List

Produce

- ❏ apples
- ❏ bananas
- ❏ broccoli
- ❏ carrots
- ❏ celery
- ❏ cherry tomatoes
- ❏ corn
- ❏ coleslaw
- ❏ cucumbers
- ❏ grapefruits
- ❏ grapes
- ❏ green beans
- ❏ green peppers
- ❏ honeydew melon
- ❏ lettuce
- ❏ mixed greens
- ❏ mushrooms
- ❏ onions
- ❏ peaches
- ❏ pear
- ❏ potatoes
- ❏ raspberries
- ❏ red onions
- ❏ red peppers
- ❏ scallions
- ❏ spinach
- ❏ squash
- ❏ strawberries
- ❏ sugar snap peas
- ❏ tomatoes
- ❏ watercress
- ❏ wax beans

Baking Products

- ❏ black pepper, ground
- ❏ blue cheese salad dressing, fat-free
- ❏ chili powder
- ❏ chili sauce
- ❏ chives
- ❏ cinnamon
- ❏ cornstarch
- ❏ cumin
- ❏ dill, fresh
- ❏ dried thyme
- ❏ dry mustard
- ❏ flour, all-purpose
- ❏ garlic powder
- ❏ garlic salt
- ❏ imitation bacon bits
- ❏ Italian salad dressing, light
- ❏ lemon juice
- ❏ nonstick cooking spray
- ❏ olive oil
- ❏ onion powder
- ❏ oriental sesame oil
- ❏ pudding, reduced-calorie chocolate-flavored
- ❏ raisins
- ❏ ranch salad dressing, fat-free
- ❏ rice vinegar
- ❏ red wine vinegar
- ❏ salsa
- ❏ salt
- ❏ sweet pickle relish
- ❏ syrup, light

- ❏ Tabasco sauce
- ❏ tomato juice
- ❏ vegetable oil
- ❏ white pepper, ground

Breads and Cereals
- ❏ bagels
- ❏ bran flakes
- ❏ bread, whole-wheat
- ❏ breadsticks
- ❏ brown rice
- ❏ English muffins
- ❏ French bread
- ❏ lasagna noodles, whole-wheat
- ❏ melba toast
- ❏ puffed rice cereal
- ❏ Raisin Bran® cereal
- ❏ rice
- ❏ saltine crackers
- ❏ wheat flakes cereal

Canned Foods
- ❏ beef broth, fat-free (1 can)
- ❏ chicken noodle soup (1 can)
- ❏ Mandarin oranges in water (1 can)
- ❏ $15^1/_2$ oz. red salmon (1 can)
- ❏ tomato sauce (1 can)

Dairy Products
- ❏ cheddar cheese, reduced-fat
- ❏ cottage cheese, lowfat
- ❏ eggs
- ❏ margarine, light
- ❏ mayonnaise, light
- ❏ milk, nonfat
- ❏ mozzarella cheese
- ❏ orange juice
- ❏ Parmesan cheese

Frozen Foods
- ❏ pancakes, frozen

Seafood and Meat
- ❏ 2 oz. chicken breast, grilled
- ❏ 2 oz. chicken breast, skinless roasted
- ❏ $1^1/_2$ to 2 lbs. chicken breast, split
- ❏ 1 lb. ground round, lean (15 percent fat or less)
- ❏ $^1/_2$ oz. ham, thinly sliced
- ❏ 1 lb. pork tenderloin
- ❏ 1 lb. 2 oz. round beef
- ❏ 6 oz. sea scallops
- ❏ 1 lb. shrimp, peeled and deveined
- ❏ $2^1/_2$ oz. shrimp, peeled and deveined

Second Week Meals and Recipes

DAY 1

Breakfast

1 cup puffed rice cereal   1 cup nonfat milk
$1/2$ medium banana, sliced

Nutritional Information: 194 calories; 1g fat (3.6% calories from fat); 10g protein; 38g carbohydrate; 2g dietary fiber; 4mg cholesterol; 127mg sodium.

Lunch

Spinach-mushroom Salad
2 cups spinach, torn   1 boiled egg, sliced
$1/4$ cup sliced mushrooms   2 tsp. imitation bacon bits
$1/4$ sliced red onion   light Italian salad dressing

Serve with:
$1/2$ cup celery sticks   1 small peach
$1/2$ cup carrot sticks   2 long breadsticks

In a medium bowl, combine spinach leaves, sliced mushrooms, sliced red onion, sliced boiled egg, imitation bacon bits and Italian salad dressing. Serves 1.

Nutritional Information: 337 calories; 12g fat (30.6% calories from fat); 14g protein; 47g carbohydrate; 9g dietary fiber; 214mg cholesterol; 619mg sodium.

Dinner

Baked Cajun Chicken
$1^1/2$ to 2 lbs. split chicken breasts $1/4$ tsp. garlic salt
2 tbsp. nonfat milk $1/8$ tsp. ground white pepper
2 tbsp. onion powder $1/8$ tsp. ground black pepper
$1/2$ tsp. dried thyme, crushed   nonstick cooking spray

Serve with:
$1/2$ cup steamed rice $1/2$ cup steamed vegetables

Rinse chicken and pat dry. Cut off skin and discard. Spray a 13″ x 9″ x 2″ baking dish with nonstick cooking spray. Arrange the chicken in the dish, meat side up. Brush lightly with milk. In small bowl, mix onion powder, thyme, garlic salt, white pepper and black pepper. Sprinkle over chicken. Bake in a 375°F oven for 45 minutes or until the chicken is cooked through. Serves 4.

Nutritional Information: 469 calories; 17g fat (33.8% calories from fat); 43g protein; 33g carbohydrate; 3g dietary fiber; 116mg cholesterol; 270mg sodium.

DAY 2

Breakfast

1 small (2-oz.) English muffin	$1/2$ medium grapefruit
1 tsp. light margarine	1 cup nonfat milk

Nutritional Information: 273 calories; 3g fat (11.2% calories from fat); 13g protein; 48g carbohydrate; 3g dietary fiber; 4mg cholesterol; 435mg sodium.

Lunch

Broiled Ham and Cheese Sandwich with Bean Salad

2 slices whole-wheat bread	$1/3$ cup green beans, steamed
$1/2$ oz. thinly sliced ham	$1/3$ cup sugar snap peas
2 tomato slices	$1/3$ cup wax beans
1 slice reduced-fat cheddar cheese	
1 tbsp. light Italian salad dressing	

Serve with: 1 small pear

Toast whole-wheat bread and then layer ham, tomato slices and cheddar cheese onto each toast slice. Place onto a nonstick baking sheet and broil until the cheese melts. For the salad, combine green beans, sugar snap peas and Italian salad dressing in a small bowl. Serves 1.

Nutritional Information: 460 calories; 10g fat (18.5% calories from fat); 27g protein; 72g carbohydrate; 14g dietary fiber; 19mg cholesterol; 991mg sodium.

Dinner

Cinnamon Apple Pork Tenderloin

1 lb. pork tenderloin
2 tbsp. cornstarch
2 tbsp. raisins

2 apples, peeled, cored and sliced
1 tsp. ground cinnamon

Serve with:

$^1/_2$ cup brown rice

1 cup green beans

Preheat the oven to 400°F. Place the pork tenderloin in a roasting pan or casserole dish with a lid. Combine the remaining ingredients in a bowl and stir. Spoon the apple mixture around the pork tenderloin. Cover and bake for 40 minutes. Remove the lid and spoon the apple mixture over the tenderloin. Return to the oven and bake 15 to 20 minutes longer until tenderloin is browned and cooked through. Serves 6.

Nutritional Information: 426 calories; 6g fat (13.3% calories from fat); 31g protein; 63g carbohydrate; 10g dietary fiber; 74mg cholesterol; 201mg sodium.

DAY 3

Breakfast

1 cup wheat flakes cereal
1 medium peach, sliced

1 cup nonfat milk

Nutritional Information: 253 calories; 3g fat (7.9% calories from fat); 18g protein; 60g carbohydrate; 27g dietary fiber; 4mg cholesterol; 127mg sodium.

Lunch

Shrimp Salad

$2^1/_2$ oz. peeled and deveined
  cooked shrimp, chopped
2 tsp. chili sauce

$^1/_2$ tsp. fresh lemon juice
2 tsp. light mayonnaise
$^1/_2$ tsp. sweet pickle relish

Serve with:

$^1/_2$ cup carrot sticks
$^1/_2$ cup celery sticks

(1) 2-oz. toasted bagel with
  1 tsp. light margarine

2 cups watercress or romaine leaves   15 grapes
   with 6 cherry tomatoes, 1 cup sliced
   cucumber and 2 tbsp. light Italian
   salad dressing

In a small bowl, combine shrimp, mayonnaise, chili sauce, lemon juice
and sweet pickle relish. Serves 1.

Nutritional Information: 464 calories; 10g Fat (19% calories from fat); 26g protein; 70g carbohydrate; 10g dietary fiber; 144mg cholesterol; 937mg sodium.

Dinner

Meat Loaf

1 egg   2 tbsp. green peppers,
$1/3$ cup onion, finely chopped   finely chopped
1 tsp. salt   1 lb. lean ground round
2 slices whole-wheat bread,   (15 percent fat or less)
   finely cubed $1/3$ cup prepared salsa
$1/2$ tsp. dry mustard

Serve with:
$1/2$ cup mashed potatoes   1 cup snap peas

Preheat oven to 400°F. Mix all ingredients well. Form into a loaf. Place
in a foil-lined 5″ x 9″ pan. Bake until done (40 to 45 minutes). Serves 4.

Nutritional Information: 459 calories; 26g fat (53.2% calories from fat); 27g protein; 25g carbohydrate; 5g dietary fiber; 139mg cholesterol; 921mg sodium.

DAY 4

Breakfast

1 small (2-oz.) bagel, toasted $3/4$ cup raspberries
   with 1 tsp. light margarine   1 cup nonfat milk

Nutritional Information: 305 calories; 4g fat (10.9% calories from fat); 15g protein; 53g carbohydrate; 8g dietary fiber; 4mg cholesterol; 475mg sodium.

Lunch

Grilled Chicken Salad
1 cup spinach leaves, torn
1/2 medium tomato, sliced
1/2 medium roasted red
  bell pepper, sliced
1/2 cup Mandarin oranges

2 oz. grilled chicken breast, sliced
2 tsp. red wine vinegar
1 tsp. olive oil
ground black pepper

Serve with:
1/2 cup reduced-calorie
  chocolate-flavored pudding

3 melba toasts

In a medium bowl, combine spinach leaves, tomato, red bell pepper, Mandarin oranges, grilled chicken breast, red wine vinegar, olive oil and freshly ground black pepper (to taste). Serves 1.

Nutritional Information: 368 calories; 9g Fat (21% calories from fat); 21g protein; 54g carbohydrate; 5g dietary fiber; 43mg cholesterol; 292mg sodium.

Dinner

Cheese Lasagna
6 oz. whole-wheat lasagna noodles
1/3 cup onions, chopped
1/3 cup red bell peppers, chopped
1/3 cup mushrooms, chopped
1 1/2 cups lowfat cottage cheese

1 cup tomato sauce
2 eggs
3 oz. mozzarella cheese, grated
2 tbsp. Parmesan cheese

Serve with:
whole-wheat dinner roll

mixed greens salad

Cook lasagna noodles in boiling water until tender. Drain and set aside. Combine tomato sauce, chopped onions, peppers and mushrooms. In a separate bowl, mix the cottage cheese, eggs and half of the Parmesan cheese. Preheat oven to 350°F. Layer half of the noodles, cottage cheese mixture and grated mozzarella cheese in an 8" x 8" casserole dish. Top with tomato sauce mix and the rest of the noodles. Sprinkle with remaining Parmesan cheese. Bake for 25 minutes and serve hot. Serves 4.

Nutritional Information: 454 calories; 9g fat (17.9% calories from fat); 30g protein; 66g carbohydrate; 9g dietary fiber; 121mg cholesterol; 1,009mg sodium.

DAY 5

Breakfast

1 cup bran flakes cereal
2 tbsp. raisins

1 cup nonfat milk

Nutritional Information: 296 calories; 2g fat (5.1% calories from fat); 14g protein; 65g carbohydrate; 9g dietary fiber; 4mg cholesterol; 474mg sodium.

Lunch

1 cup canned chicken noodle soup
1 cup broccoli florets with
  2 tbsp. fat-free ranch dressing
2-inch wedge honeydew melon

2 oz.-cube of reduced-fat cheddar
  cheese
8 lowfat saltines

Nutritional Information: 388 calories; 10g fat (23.1% calories from fat); 20g protein; 57g carbohydrate; 6g dietary fiber; 30mg cholesterol; 2,667mg sodium.

Dinner

Steamed Shrimp and Scallops

1 lb. shrimp, peeled and deveined
6 oz. sea scallops
$1/4$ cup orange juice
2 tsp. rice vinegar
1 tbsp. oriental sesame oil
$1/2$ tsp. dry mustard

$1/2$ tsp. salt
$1/4$ tsp. freshly ground black pepper
2 scallions, thinly sliced
1 tbsp. fresh dill, chopped
1 tsp. chives, chopped
4 lettuce leaves

Serve with:
1 corn on the cob
1 roasted potato

1 cup green beans

Arrange the shrimp and scallops on a plate in a steamer basket. Sprinkle with 1 teaspoon each of the orange juice and rice vinegar. Place steamer over boiling water in a wok or large skillet and cover. Cook 7 to 8 minutes until the shrimp are cooked through. Meanwhile, stir together the remaining orange juice, rice vinegar, sesame oil, mustard, salt and pepper in a medium bowl. Mix in scallions, dill and chives. Transfer hot seafood to the bowl with the vinaigrette and toss to coat well. Serve warm on lettuce-lined plates. Garnish with chopped pimento, if desired. Serves 4.

Nutritional Information: 483 calories; 8g Fat (15% calories from fat); 40g protein; 66g carbohydrate; 11g dietary fiber; 187mg cholesterol; 668mg sodium.

DAY 6

Breakfast

2 frozen pancakes
2 tsp. light syrup

$^1/_2$ medium grapefruit
1 cup nonfat milk

Nutritional Information: 288 calories; 3g fat (9.1% calories from fat); 13g protein; 53g carbohydrate; 3g dietary fiber; 11mg cholesterol; 493mg sodium.

Lunch

2 oz. skinless roast chicken
  breast, cut into strips
$^1/_2$ cup cooked brown rice with
  1 tsp. light margarine
$^1/_2$ cup each steamed whole green
  beans and julienne carrots with
  $^1/_2$ tsp. fresh lemon juice

2 cups mixed field green salad with
  1 tbsp. fat-free blue cheese dressing
1 slice French bread, toasted, with
  1 tsp. light margarine
1 small apple

Nutritional Information: 515 calories; 11g fat (18.1% calories from fat); 27g protein; 81g carbohydrate; 14g dietary fiber; 48mg cholesterol; 543mg sodium.

Dinner

Salmon Cakes

(1) 15$^1/_2$-oz. can red salmon, drained
  (2 cups flaked)
$^1/_4$ cup red pepper or canned
  pimiento, diced
6 unsalted-top saltine crackers,
  crushed

1 tsp. onion powder
4 drops Tabasco sauce
3 tbsp. light salad dressing
  or mayonnaise
nonstick cooking spray

Serve with:
1 cup coleslaw

1 breadstick

Remove skin from fish. Combine all ingredients in a medium bowl, mashing salmon bones with a fork. Shape into 4 cakes. Spray a skillet with nonstick cooking spray and heat over medium heat. Cook salmon cakes, turning once, until lightly browned on each side. Serves 2.

Nutritional Information: 466 calories; 16g fat (30.8% calories from fat); 47g protein; 35g carbohydrate; 4g dietary fiber; 128mg cholesterol; 419mg sodium.

DAY 7

Breakfast

2 slices whole-wheat bread, toasted
2 tsp. light margarine
$^3/_4$ oz. Raisin Bran® cereal

1 cup strawberries
$^1/_2$ cup nonfat milk

Nutritional Information: 324 calories; 7g fat (18.6% calories from fat); 13g protein; 58g carbohydrate; 9g dietary fiber; 2mg cholesterol; 607mg sodium.

Lunch

Arby's Junior Roast Beef Sandwich®
1 cup coleslaw

1 cup mixed melon balls

Nutritional Information: 497 calories; 18g fat (32.2% calories from fat); 24g protein; 64g carbohydrate; 4g dietary fiber; 37mg cholesterol; 1,383mg sodium.

Dinner

Texas Round Steak

$^1/_2$ cup all-purpose flour
$1^1/_2$ tsp. chili powder
1 lb. 2 oz. round beef,
   cut into 6 pieces
$^1/_2$ cup fresh green peppers
1 cup fat-free beef broth
1 tsp. chili power

1 tsp. salt
1 tbsp. vegetable oil
$^1/_2$ cup chopped onions
$^1/_2$ cup tomato juice
$^1/_4$ tsp. garlic powder
$^1/_3$ tsp. ground cumin

Serve with:

1 cup roasted potatoes

1 cup sautéed squash

Blend flour, salt and chili powder well and place in pie pan. Dredge the meat in the flour mixture (use about half of the mixture). Place vegetable oil in a heavy frying pan and heat to frying temperature over moderate heat. Add meat and brown on both sides. Transfer steaks to a 1$^1/_2$-quart casserole. Fry peppers and onions over moderate heat in the pan in which the meat was browned, stirring frequently. Remove vegetables with a slotted spoon and spread over meat. Pour out any remaining fat. Add beef broth to frying pan and cook and stir over moderate heat to loosen the brown particles remaining in the pan. Add remaining ingredients to broth. Mix well and pour over meat. Stir the meat and vegetables lightly with a fork to distribute the broth and vegetables. Cover tightly and bake at 325°F for about 1 to 1$^1/_2$ hours, or until the meat is tender. Serve some of the sauté with each piece of steak. Serves 6.

Nutritional Information: 509 calories; 20g fat (34.5% calories from fat); 34g protein; 50g carbohydrate; 6g dietary fiber; 76mg cholesterol; 1,049mg sodium.

HEALTHY SNACK OPTIONS
(**Note:** You will need to add the ingredients for these items to the grocery lists.)

- 30 small pretzel sticks: 90 calories
- 1 banana-chocolate whip (combine 1 cup fat-free milk, 1 small banana, a squeeze of chocolate syrup and a handful of ice cubes in a blender): 150 calories
- 3 cups air-popped popcorn sprinkled with 1 tbsp. Parmesan cheese: 120 calories
- Snack plate: 25 red grapes, 3 tablespoons feta cheese, 6 crackers: 200 calories

DESSERT AND SNACK RECIPES
Apple Crunch Bar
2 cups all-purpose flour
$^1/_2$ cup brown sugar substitute
$^1/_2$ cup brown sugar, firmly packed
$^1/_4$ cup butter, softened
1 tsp. baking soda
1 tsp. ground cinnamon
$^1/_4$ tsp. ground nutmeg
$^1/_8$ tsp. salt

1 tsp. vanilla extract
8 oz. plain lowfat yogurt
1 medium egg
2 cups Granny Smith apples, chopped
$^1/_2$ cup raisins, seedless
$^1/_4$ cup chopped walnuts
1 tbsp. sugar
nonstick cooking spray

Combine flour, brown sugar, brown sugar substitute and butter in a bowl, beating well with an electric mixer at medium speed. Reserve 2 cups of the flour mixture and set aside. Add baking soda, cinnamon, nutmeg and salt to the remaining flour mixture and beat well. Add vanilla, yogurt and egg and beat well. Stir in apples and raisins. Press 2 cups of the reserved flour mixture (will be very dry) into the bottom of a 9" x 13" x 2" baking pan well coated with cooking spray. Sprinkle walnuts over flour mixture. Spread apple mixture over prepared crust. Bake at 350°F for 35 to 40 minutes, or until browned. Cool completely in a pan on a wire rack. Sprinkle with remaining tablespoon of sugar before cutting. Serves 16.

Nutritional Information: 105 calories; 3g fat (26.4% calories from fat); 2g protein; 17g carbohydrate; 1g dietary fiber; 15mg cholesterol; 95mg sodium.

Fresh Fruit Salsa with Sweet Tortilla Chips

(**Note:** This recipe is ideal to prepare a day or two ahead of time and refrigerate. Store the chips in a closeable plastic storage bag.)

2 pints strawberries
4 kiwis, peeled and diced
1 Granny Smith apple, diced
3 tbsp. orange all-fruit spread
1 orange rind, grated
1 pint fresh blackberries, diced
1 pint fresh raspberries, diced

1 tbsp. fresh finely chopped mint
$1/2$ cup and 1 tbsp. Splenda®
  Granular
(6) 6-inch reduced-fat flour tortillas
1 tsp. sugar
$1/2$ cup hot water

Preheat oven to 225°F. Remove stems from the strawberries and dice. In a large bowl, mix strawberries, kiwis, Granny Smith apple, orange fruit spread, orange rind, blackberries, raspberries and mint. Sprinkle on $1/2$ cup of the Splenda® and toss lightly to blend. In a small bowl, mix sugar and water. Brush the tortillas with the sugar water. Cut flour tortillas in half and then each half into 6 pieces. Place on an ungreased cookie sheet and bake for 10 to 15 minutes. Cool for 5 minutes and dust with remaining Splenda®. Serves 12. (Serving size: 6 chips, $1/2$-cup fruit mixture.)

Nutritional Information: 126 calories; 1g fat (8.8% calories from fat); 1g protein; 28g carbohydrate; 7g dietary fiber; 0mg cholesterol; 167mg sodium.

Watermelon and Kiwi on a Skewer

1/4 cup sliced strawberries
1/2 cup vanilla lowfat
  sugar-free yogurt
1 tbsp. lowfat cream cheese

1 tsp. fresh lemon juice
24 watermelon balls
2 kiwi fruit, peeled and cut
  into 24 pieces

Place strawberries, yogurt, cream cheese and lemon juice into a blender and process until smooth to make a sauce. Cover and chill. Thread 2 watermelon balls and 2 kiwi fruit pieces each onto 12 skewers. Serve with the sauce. Serves 4.

Nutritional Information: 82 calories; 2g fat (15.3% calories from fat); 2g protein; 16g carbohydrate; 2g dietary fiber; 4mg cholesterol; 42mg sodium.

Lowfat Granola with Dried Fruit

1 cup boiling water
1/4 cup dried cranberries
(1) 6-oz. pkg. dried mixed
  tropical fruit
2 tbsp. packed brown sugar
3 cups regular oats

1/4 cup sliced almonds
1/4 cup chopped pecans
1/4 cup unsweetened coconut flakes
1/2 tsp. ground cinnamon
1/2 tsp. vanilla
nonstick cooking spray

Preheat oven to 300°F. In a bowl, combine water, cranberries, mixed tropical fruit and brown sugar and let stand for 15 minutes. In a large bowl, combine oats and remaining ingredients, and then stir in the fruit mixture. Coat two cookie sheets with nonstick cooking spray and spread mixture to a depth of about 1/2 inch. Bake at 300°F for 1 hour, stirring every 15 minutes. Cool to room temperature and store in an airtight container. Serves 12. (Serving size: 1/2 cup.)

Nutritional Information: 237 calories; 7g fat (23.8% calories from fat); 8g protein; 39g carbohydrate; 6g dietary fiber; 0mg cholesterol; 9mg sodium.

Death by Chocolate

(**Note:** This makes a huge dessert for company. For smaller get-togethers, store half of the brownies for later use and halve the other ingredients accordingly.)

1 box reduced-fat Brownie Mix
2 large boxes sugar-free
  vanilla pudding
4 cups nonfat milk

1 cup half and half, fat-free
12 oz. Cool Whip Lite®
1 tbsp. mini-chocolate chips

Make and bake brownies according to package directions and cool. If desired, drizzle 2 to 3 tablespoons of strong coffee over the top. Break or cut into bite-sized pieces. Mix pudding with skim milk and half and half. Layer three times in order in a trifle dish (brownies, pudding, Cool Whip®) and put 1 tablespoon of the chocolate chips on top. Serves 24.

Nutritional Information: 152 calories; 4g fat (21.9% calories from fat); 3g protein; 26g carbohydrate; 1g dietary fiber; 1mg cholesterol; 157mg sodium.

Grilled Banana Split

1 whole banana
$^1/_2$ tbsp. chocolate chips

1 tbsp. crushed pineapple
2 tbsp. miniature marshmallows

Slice the banana length-wise (leave the peel on) and sprinkle chocolate chips and marshmallows over the top. Place under broiler for 2 to 3 minutes to melt the chips and marshmallows. Remove from the oven and sprinkle pineapple on top. Eat directly out of the peel. Serves 1.

Nutritional Information: 171 calories; 3g fat (13.7% calories from fat); 2g protein; 38g carbohydrate; 3g dietary fiber; 0mg cholesterol; 4mg sodium.

Member Survey

Please answer the following questions to help your leader plan your First Place 4 Health meetings so that your needs might be met in this session. Give this form to your leader at the first group meeting.

Name _____ Birth date _____

Please list those who live in your household.

Name	Relationship	Age

What church do you attend? _____

Are you interested in receiving more information about our church?

❒ Yes   ❒ No

Occupation _____

What talent or area of expertise would you be willing to share with our class?

_____

Why did you join First Place 4 Health?

_____

With notice, would you be willing to lead a Bible study discussion one week?

❒ Yes   ❒ No

Are you comfortable praying out loud? _____

If the assistant leader were absent, would you be willing to assist in weighing in members and possibly evaluating the Live It Trackers?

❒ Yes   ❒ No

Any other comments:

_____
_____

Personal Weight and Measurement Record

Week	Weight	+ or -	Goal this Session	Pounds to goal
1				
2				
3				
4				
5				
6				
7				
8				
9				
10				
11				
12				

Beginning Measurements

Waist _____ Hips _____ Thighs _____ Chest _____

Ending Measurements

Waist _____ Hips _____ Thighs _____ Chest _____

First Place 4 Health
Prayer Partner

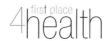

Scripture Verse to Memorize for Week Two:

Not to us, O Lord, not to us but to your name be the glory,
because of your love and faithfulness.

Psalm 115:1

Date: _____

Name: _____

Home Phone: (_____) _____

Work Phone: (_____) _____

Email: _____

Personal Prayer Concerns:

_____

_____

_____

_____

_____

_____

_____

This form is for prayer requests that are personal to you and your journey in First Place 4 Health. Please complete this form and have it ready to turn in when you arrive at your group meeting.

First Place 4 Health
Prayer Partner

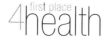

CELEBRATE
SUCCESS
Week
3

Date: _____

Name: _____

Home Phone: ( ) _____

Work Phone: ( ) _____

Email: _____

Personal Prayer Concerns:

_____

_____

_____

_____

_____

_____

_____

This form is for prayer requests that are personal to you and your journey in First Place 4 Health. Please complete this form and have it ready to turn in when you arrive at your group meeting.

First Place 4 Health
Prayer Partner

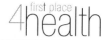

SCRIPTURE VERSE TO MEMORIZE FOR WEEK SIX:
I say to myself, "The LORD is my portion;
therefore I will wait for him."

LAMENTATIONS 3:24

Date: _____

Name: _____

Home Phone: (_____) _____

Work Phone: (_____) _____

Email: _____

Personal Prayer Concerns:

_____

_____

_____

_____

_____

_____

_____

This form is for prayer requests that are personal to you and your journey in First Place 4 Health. Please complete this form and have it ready to turn in when you arrive at your group meeting.

First Place 4 Health
Prayer Partner

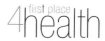

SCRIPTURE VERSE TO MEMORIZE FOR WEEK SEVEN:

Do not defile the land where you live and where I dwell,
for I, the LORD, dwell among the Israelites.

NUMBERS 35:34

Date: _____

Name: _____

Home Phone: (_____) _____

Work Phone: (_____) _____

Email: _____

Personal Prayer Concerns:

_____

_____

_____

_____

_____

_____

_____

This form is for prayer requests that are personal to you and your journey in First Place 4 Health. Please complete this form and have it ready to turn in when you arrive at your group meeting.

First Place 4 Health
Prayer Partner

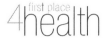

SCRIPTURE VERSE TO MEMORIZE FOR WEEK EIGHT:
*Speak to one another with psalms, hymns and spiritual songs.
Sing and make music in your heart to the Lord.*
EPHESIANS 5:19

Date: _____

Name: _____

Home Phone: (_____) _____

Work Phone: (_____) _____

Email: _____

Personal Prayer Concerns:

_____

_____

_____

_____

_____

_____

_____

This form is for prayer requests that are personal to you and your journey in First Place 4 Health. Please complete this form and have it ready to turn in when you arrive at your group meeting.

Live It Tracker

Name: _____ Loss/gain: _____ lbs.

Date: _____ Week #: _____ Calorie Range: _____ My food goal for next week: _____

Activity Level: None, < 30 min/day, 30-60 min/day, 60+ min/day My activity goal for next week: _____

Group	Daily Calories							
	1300-1400	1500-1600	1700-1800	1900-2000	2100-2200	2300-2400	2500-2600	2700-2800
Fruits	1.5-2 c.	1.5-2 c.	1.5-2 c.	2-2.5 c.	2-2.5 c.	2.5-3.5 c.	3.5-4.5 c.	3.5-4.5 c.
Vegetables	1.5-2 c.	2-2.5 c.	2.5-3 c.	2.5-3 c.	3-3.5 c.	3.5-4.5 c.	4.5-5 c.	4.5-5 c.
Grains	5 oz-eq.	5-6 oz-eq.	6-7 oz-eq.	6-7 oz-eq.	7-8 oz-eq.	8-9 oz-eq.	9-10 oz-eq.	10-11 oz-eq.
Meat & Beans	4 oz-eq.	5 oz-eq.	5-5.5 oz-eq.	5.5-6.5 oz-eq.	6.5-7 oz-eq.	7-7.5 oz-eq.	7-7.5 oz-eq.	7.5-8 oz-eq.
Milk	2-3 c.	3 c.	3 c.	3 c.	3 c.	3 c.	3 c.	3 c.
Healthy Oils	4 tsp.	5 tsp.	5 tsp.	6 tsp.	6 tsp.	7 tsp.	8 tsp.	8 tsp.

Day/Date:

Breakfast: _____ Lunch: _____

Dinner: _____ Snack: _____

Group	Fruits	Vegetables	Grains	Meat & Beans	Milk	Oils
Goal Amount						
Estimate Your Total						
Increase ⇧ or Decrease? ⇩						

Physical Activity: _____ Spiritual Activity: _____

Steps/Miles/Minutes: _____ _____

Day/Date:

Breakfast: _____ Lunch: _____

Dinner: _____ Snack: _____

Group	Fruits	Vegetables	Grains	Meat & Beans	Milk	Oils
Goal Amount						
Estimate Your Total						
Increase ⇧ or Decrease? ⇩						

Physical Activity: _____ Spiritual Activity: _____

Steps/Miles/Minutes: _____ _____

Day/Date:

Breakfast: _____ Lunch: _____

Dinner: _____ Snack: _____

Group	Fruits	Vegetables	Grains	Meat & Beans	Milk	Oils
Goal Amount						
Estimate Your Total						
Increase ⇧ or Decrease? ⇩						

Physical Activity: _____ Spiritual Activity: _____

Steps/Miles/Minutes: _____

Day/Date: _____

Breakfast: _____ Lunch: _____

Dinner: _____ Snack: _____

Group	Fruits	Vegetables	Grains	Meat & Beans	Milk	Oils
Goal Amount						
Estimate Your Total						
Increase ⇧ or Decrease? ⇩						

Physical Activity: _____ Spiritual Activity: _____

Steps/Miles/Minutes: _____ _____

Day/Date: _____

Breakfast: _____ Lunch: _____

Dinner: _____ Snack: _____

Group	Fruits	Vegetables	Grains	Meat & Beans	Milk	Oils
Goal Amount						
Estimate Your Total						
Increase ⇧ or Decrease? ⇩						

Physical Activity: _____ Spiritual Activity: _____

Steps/Miles/Minutes: _____ _____

Day/Date: _____

Breakfast: _____ Lunch: _____

Dinner: _____ Snack: _____

Group	Fruits	Vegetables	Grains	Meat & Beans	Milk	Oils
Goal Amount						
Estimate Your Total						
Increase ⇧ or Decrease? ⇩						

Physical Activity: _____ Spiritual Activity: _____

Steps/Miles/Minutes: _____ _____

Day/Date: _____

Breakfast: _____ Lunch: _____

Dinner: _____ Snack: _____

Group	Fruits	Vegetables	Grains	Meat & Beans	Milk	Oils
Goal Amount						
Estimate Your Total						
Increase ⇧ or Decrease? ⇩						

Physical Activity: _____ Spiritual Activity: _____

Steps/Miles/Minutes: _____ _____

Live It Tracker

Name: _____ Loss/gain: _____ lbs.

Date: _____ Week #: _____ Calorie Range: _____ My food goal for next week: _____

Activity Level: None, < 30 min/day, 30-60 min/day, 60+ min/day My activity goal for next week: _____

Group	Daily Calories							
	1300-1400	1500-1600	1700-1800	1900-2000	2100-2200	2300-2400	2500-2600	2700-2800
Fruits	1.5-2 c.	1.5-2 c.	1.5-2 c.	2-2.5 c.	2-2.5 c.	2.5-3.5 c.	3.5-4.5 c.	3.5-4.5 c.
Vegetables	1.5-2 c.	2-2.5 c.	2.5-3 c.	2.5-3 c.	3-3.5 c.	3.5-4.5 c.	4.5-5 c.	4.5-5 c.
Grains	5 oz-eq.	5-6 oz-eq.	6-7 oz-eq.	6-7 oz-eq.	7-8 oz-eq.	8-9 oz-eq.	9-10 oz-eq.	10-11 oz-eq.
Meat & Beans	4 oz-eq.	5 oz-eq.	5-5.5 oz-eq.	5.5-6.5 oz-eq.	6.5-7 oz-eq.	7-7.5 oz-eq.	7-7.5 oz-eq.	7.5-8 oz-eq.
Milk	2-3 c.	3 c.	3 c.	3 c.	3 c.	3 c.	3 c.	3 c.
Healthy Oils	4 tsp.	5 tsp.	5 tsp.	6 tsp.	6 tsp.	7 tsp.	8 tsp.	8 tsp.

Day/Date: _____

Breakfast: _____ Lunch: _____

Dinner: _____ Snack: _____

Group	Fruits	Vegetables	Grains	Meat & Beans	Milk	Oils
Goal Amount						
Estimate Your Total						
Increase ⬆ or Decrease? ⬇						

Physical Activity: _____ Spiritual Activity: _____

Steps/Miles/Minutes: _____

Day/Date: _____

Breakfast: _____ Lunch: _____

Dinner: _____ Snack: _____

Group	Fruits	Vegetables	Grains	Meat & Beans	Milk	Oils
Goal Amount						
Estimate Your Total						
Increase ⬆ or Decrease? ⬇						

Physical Activity: _____ Spiritual Activity: _____

Steps/Miles/Minutes: _____

Day/Date: _____

Breakfast: _____ Lunch: _____

Dinner: _____ Snack: _____

Group	Fruits	Vegetables	Grains	Meat & Beans	Milk	Oils
Goal Amount						
Estimate Your Total						
Increase ⬆ or Decrease? ⬇						

Physical Activity: _____ Spiritual Activity: _____

Steps/Miles/Minutes: _____

Day/Date: _____

Breakfast: _____   Lunch: _____

Dinner: _____   Snack: _____

Group	Fruits	Vegetables	Grains	Meat & Beans	Milk	Oils
Goal Amount						
Estimate Your Total						
Increase ⇧ or Decrease? ⇩						

Physical Activity: _____   Spiritual Activity: _____

Steps/Miles/Minutes: _____   _____

Day/Date: _____

Breakfast: _____   Lunch: _____

Dinner: _____   Snack: _____

Group	Fruits	Vegetables	Grains	Meat & Beans	Milk	Oils
Goal Amount						
Estimate Your Total						
Increase ⇧ or Decrease? ⇩						

Physical Activity: _____   Spiritual Activity: _____

Steps/Miles/Minutes: _____   _____

Day/Date: _____

Breakfast: _____   Lunch: _____

Dinner: _____   Snack: _____

Group	Fruits	Vegetables	Grains	Meat & Beans	Milk	Oils
Goal Amount						
Estimate Your Total						
Increase ⇧ or Decrease? ⇩						

Physical Activity: _____   Spiritual Activity: _____

Steps/Miles/Minutes: _____   _____

Day/Date: _____

Breakfast: _____   Lunch: _____

Dinner: _____   Snack: _____

Group	Fruits	Vegetables	Grains	Meat & Beans	Milk	Oils
Goal Amount						
Estimate Your Total						
Increase ⇧ or Decrease? ⇩						

Physical Activity: _____   Spiritual Activity: _____

Steps/Miles/Minutes: _____   _____

Live It Tracker

Name: _____ Loss/gain: _____ lbs.

Date: _____ Week #: _____ Calorie Range: _____ My food goal for next week: _____

Activity Level: None, < 30 min/day, 30-60 min/day, 60+ min/day   My activity goal for next week: _____

Group	Daily Calories							
	1300-1400	1500-1600	1700-1800	1900-2000	2100-2200	2300-2400	2500-2600	2700-2800
Fruits	1.5-2 c.	1.5-2 c.	1.5-2 c.	2-2.5 c.	2-2.5 c.	2.5-3.5 c.	3.5-4.5 c.	3.5-4.5 c.
Vegetables	1.5-2 c.	2-2.5 c.	2.5-3 c.	2.5-3 c.	3-3.5 c.	3.5-4.5 c.	4.5-5 c.	4.5-5 c.
Grains	5 oz-eq.	5-6 oz-eq.	6-7 oz-eq.	6-7 oz-eq.	7-8 oz-eq.	8-9 oz-eq.	9-10 oz-eq.	10-11 oz-eq.
Meat & Beans	4 oz-eq.	5 oz-eq.	5-5.5 oz-eq.	5.5-6.5 oz-eq.	6.5-7 oz-eq.	7-7.5 oz-eq.	7-7.5 oz-eq.	7.5-8 oz-eq.
Milk	2-3 c.	3 c.	3 c.	3 c.	3 c.	3 c.	3 c.	3 c.
Healthy Oils	4 tsp.	5 tsp.	5 tsp.	6 tsp.	6 tsp.	7 tsp.	8 tsp.	8 tsp.

Day/Date:

Breakfast: _____   Lunch: _____

Dinner: _____   Snack: _____

Group	Fruits	Vegetables	Grains	Meat & Beans	Milk	Oils
Goal Amount						
Estimate Your Total						
Increase ⇧ or Decrease? ⇩						

Physical Activity: _____   Spiritual Activity: _____

Steps/Miles/Minutes: _____

Day/Date:

Breakfast: _____   Lunch: _____

Dinner: _____   Snack: _____

Group	Fruits	Vegetables	Grains	Meat & Beans	Milk	Oils
Goal Amount						
Estimate Your Total						
Increase ⇧ or Decrease? ⇩						

Physical Activity: _____   Spiritual Activity: _____

Steps/Miles/Minutes: _____

Day/Date:

Breakfast: _____   Lunch: _____

Dinner: _____   Snack: _____

Group	Fruits	Vegetables	Grains	Meat & Beans	Milk	Oils
Goal Amount						
Estimate Your Total						
Increase ⇧ or Decrease? ⇩						

Physical Activity: _____   Spiritual Activity: _____

Steps/Miles/Minutes: _____

Day/Date: _____

Breakfast: _____ Lunch: _____

Dinner: _____ Snack: _____

Group	Fruits	Vegetables	Grains	Meat & Beans	Milk	Oils
Goal Amount						
Estimate Your Total						
Increase ⇧ or Decrease? ⇩						

Physical Activity: _____ Spiritual Activity: _____

Steps/Miles/Minutes: _____ _____

Day/Date: _____

Breakfast: _____ Lunch: _____

Dinner: _____ Snack: _____

Group	Fruits	Vegetables	Grains	Meat & Beans	Milk	Oils
Goal Amount						
Estimate Your Total						
Increase ⇧ or Decrease? ⇩						

Physical Activity: _____ Spiritual Activity: _____

Steps/Miles/Minutes: _____ _____

Day/Date: _____

Breakfast: _____ Lunch: _____

Dinner: _____ Snack: _____

Group	Fruits	Vegetables	Grains	Meat & Beans	Milk	Oils
Goal Amount						
Estimate Your Total						
Increase ⇧ or Decrease? ⇩						

Physical Activity: _____ Spiritual Activity: _____

Steps/Miles/Minutes: _____ _____

Day/Date: _____

Breakfast: _____ Lunch: _____

Dinner: _____ Snack: _____

Group	Fruits	Vegetables	Grains	Meat & Beans	Milk	Oils
Goal Amount						
Estimate Your Total						
Increase ⇧ or Decrease? ⇩						

Physical Activity: _____ Spiritual Activity: _____

Steps/Miles/Minutes: _____ _____

Live It Tracker

Name: _____ Loss/gain: _____ lbs.

Date: _____ Week #: ____ Calorie Range: _____ My food goal for next week: _____

Activity Level: None, < 30 min/day, 30-60 min/day, 60+ min/day My activity goal for next week: _____

Group	Daily Calories							
	1300-1400	1500-1600	1700-1800	1900-2000	2100-2200	2300-2400	2500-2600	2700-2800
Fruits	1.5-2 c.	1.5-2 c.	1.5-2 c.	2-2.5 c.	2-2.5 c.	2.5-3.5 c.	3.5-4.5 c.	3.5-4.5 c.
Vegetables	1.5-2 c.	2-2.5 c.	2.5-3 c.	2.5-3 c.	3-3.5 c.	3.5-4.5 c.	4.5-5 c.	4.5-5 c.
Grains	5 oz-eq.	5-6 oz-eq.	6-7 oz-eq.	6-7 oz-eq.	7-8 oz-eq.	8-9 oz-eq.	9-10 oz-eq.	10-11 oz-eq.
Meat & Beans	4 oz-eq.	5 oz-eq.	5-5.5 oz-eq.	5.5-6.5 oz-eq.	6.5-7 oz-eq.	7-7.5 oz-eq.	7-7.5 oz-eq.	7.5-8 oz-eq.
Milk	2-3 c.	3 c.	3 c.	3 c.	3 c.	3 c.	3 c.	3 c.
Healthy Oils	4 tsp.	5 tsp.	5 tsp.	6 tsp.	6 tsp.	7 tsp.	8 tsp.	8 tsp.

Day/Date:

Breakfast: _____ Lunch: _____

Dinner: _____ Snack: _____

Group	Fruits	Vegetables	Grains	Meat & Beans	Milk	Oils
Goal Amount						
Estimate Your Total						
Increase ⇧ or Decrease? ⇩						

Physical Activity: _____ Spiritual Activity: _____

Steps/Miles/Minutes: _____

Day/Date:

Breakfast: _____ Lunch: _____

Dinner: _____ Snack: _____

Group	Fruits	Vegetables	Grains	Meat & Beans	Milk	Oils
Goal Amount						
Estimate Your Total						
Increase ⇧ or Decrease? ⇩						

Physical Activity: _____ Spiritual Activity: _____

Steps/Miles/Minutes: _____

Day/Date:

Breakfast: _____ Lunch: _____

Dinner: _____ Snack: _____

Group	Fruits	Vegetables	Grains	Meat & Beans	Milk	Oils
Goal Amount						
Estimate Your Total						
Increase ⇧ or Decrease? ⇩						

Physical Activity: _____ Spiritual Activity: _____

Steps/Miles/Minutes: _____

Day/Date:

Breakfast: _____   Lunch: _____

Dinner: _____   Snack: _____

Group	Fruits	Vegetables	Grains	Meat & Beans	Milk	Oils
Goal Amount						
Estimate Your Total						
Increase ⇧ or Decrease? ⇩						

Physical Activity: _____   Spiritual Activity: _____

Steps/Miles/Minutes: _____

Day/Date:

Breakfast: _____   Lunch: _____

Dinner: _____   Snack: _____

Group	Fruits	Vegetables	Grains	Meat & Beans	Milk	Oils
Goal Amount						
Estimate Your Total						
Increase ⇧ or Decrease? ⇩						

Physical Activity: _____   Spiritual Activity: _____

Steps/Miles/Minutes: _____

Day/Date:

Breakfast: _____   Lunch: _____

Dinner: _____   Snack: _____

Group	Fruits	Vegetables	Grains	Meat & Beans	Milk	Oils
Goal Amount						
Estimate Your Total						
Increase ⇧ or Decrease? ⇩						

Physical Activity: _____   Spiritual Activity: _____

Steps/Miles/Minutes: _____

Day/Date:

Breakfast: _____   Lunch: _____

Dinner: _____   Snack: _____

Group	Fruits	Vegetables	Grains	Meat & Beans	Milk	Oils
Goal Amount						
Estimate Your Total						
Increase ⇧ or Decrease? ⇩						

Physical Activity: _____   Spiritual Activity: _____

Steps/Miles/Minutes: _____

Live It Tracker

Name: _____ Loss/gain: _____ lbs.

Date: _____ Week #: _____ Calorie Range: _____ My food goal for next week: _____

Activity Level: None, < 30 min/day, 30-60 min/day, 60+ min/day My activity goal for next week: _____

Group	Daily Calories							
	1300-1400	1500-1600	1700-1800	1900-2000	2100-2200	2300-2400	2500-2600	2700-2800
Fruits	1.5-2 c.	1.5-2 c.	1.5-2 c.	2-2.5 c.	2-2.5 c.	2.5-3.5 c.	3.5-4.5 c.	3.5-4.5 c.
Vegetables	1.5-2 c.	2-2.5 c.	2.5-3 c.	2.5-3 c.	3-3.5 c.	3.5-4.5 c.	4.5-5 c.	4.5-5 c.
Grains	5 oz-eq.	5-6 oz-eq.	6-7 oz-eq.	6-7 oz-eq.	7-8 oz-eq.	8-9 oz-eq.	9-10 oz-eq.	10-11 oz-eq.
Meat & Beans	4 oz-eq.	5 oz-eq.	5-5.5 oz-eq.	5.5-6.5 oz-eq.	6.5-7 oz-eq.	7-7.5 oz-eq.	7-7.5 oz-eq.	7.5-8 oz-eq.
Milk	2-3 c.	3 c.	3 c.	3 c.	3 c.	3 c.	3 c.	3 c.
Healthy Oils	4 tsp.	5 tsp.	5 tsp.	6 tsp.	6 tsp.	7 tsp.	8 tsp.	8 tsp.

Day/Date:

Breakfast: _____ Lunch: _____

Dinner: _____ Snack: _____

Group	Fruits	Vegetables	Grains	Meat & Beans	Milk	Oils
Goal Amount						
Estimate Your Total						
Increase ⇧ or Decrease? ⇩						

Physical Activity: _____ Spiritual Activity: _____

Steps/Miles/Minutes: _____

Day/Date:

Breakfast: _____ Lunch: _____

Dinner: _____ Snack: _____

Group	Fruits	Vegetables	Grains	Meat & Beans	Milk	Oils
Goal Amount						
Estimate Your Total						
Increase ⇧ or Decrease? ⇩						

Physical Activity: _____ Spiritual Activity: _____

Steps/Miles/Minutes: _____

Day/Date:

Breakfast: _____ Lunch: _____

Dinner: _____ Snack: _____

Group	Fruits	Vegetables	Grains	Meat & Beans	Milk	Oils
Goal Amount						
Estimate Your Total						
Increase ⇧ or Decrease? ⇩						

Physical Activity: _____ Spiritual Activity: _____

Steps/Miles/Minutes: _____

Day/Date: ____

Breakfast: _____ Lunch: _____

Dinner: _____ Snack: _____

Group	Fruits	Vegetables	Grains	Meat & Beans	Milk	Oils
Goal Amount						
Estimate Your Total						
Increase ⇧ or Decrease? ⇩						

Physical Activity: _____ Spiritual Activity: _____

Steps/Miles/Minutes: _____ _____

Day/Date: ____

Breakfast: _____ Lunch: _____

Dinner: _____ Snack: _____

Group	Fruits	Vegetables	Grains	Meat & Beans	Milk	Oils
Goal Amount						
Estimate Your Total						
Increase ⇧ or Decrease? ⇩						

Physical Activity: _____ Spiritual Activity: _____

Steps/Miles/Minutes: _____ _____

Day/Date: ____

Breakfast: _____ Lunch: _____

Dinner: _____ Snack: _____

Group	Fruits	Vegetables	Grains	Meat & Beans	Milk	Oils
Goal Amount						
Estimate Your Total						
Increase ⇧ or Decrease? ⇩						

Physical Activity: _____ Spiritual Activity: _____

Steps/Miles/Minutes: _____ _____

Day/Date: ____

Breakfast: _____ Lunch: _____

Dinner: _____ Snack: _____

Group	Fruits	Vegetables	Grains	Meat & Beans	Milk	Oils
Goal Amount						
Estimate Your Total						
Increase ⇧ or Decrease? ⇩						

Physical Activity: _____ Spiritual Activity: _____

Steps/Miles/Minutes: _____ _____

Live It Tracker

Name: _____ Loss/gain: _____ lbs.

Date: _____ Week #: _____ Calorie Range: _____ My food goal for next week: _____

Activity Level: None, < 30 min/day, 30-60 min/day, 60+ min/day My activity goal for next week: _____

Group	Daily Calories							
	1300-1400	1500-1600	1700-1800	1900-2000	2100-2200	2300-2400	2500-2600	2700-2800
Fruits	1.5-2 c.	1.5-2 c.	1.5-2 c.	2-2.5 c.	2-2.5 c.	2.5-3.5 c.	3.5-4.5 c.	3.5-4.5 c.
Vegetables	1.5-2 c.	2-2.5 c.	2.5-3 c.	2.5-3 c.	3-3.5 c.	3.5-4.5 c.	4.5-5 c.	4.5-5 c.
Grains	5 oz-eq.	5-6 oz-eq.	6-7 oz-eq.	6-7 oz-eq.	7-8 oz-eq.	8-9 oz-eq.	9-10 oz-eq.	10-11 oz-eq.
Meat & Beans	4 oz-eq.	5 oz-eq.	5-5.5 oz-eq.	5.5-6.5 oz-eq.	6.5-7 oz-eq.	7-7.5 oz-eq.	7-7.5 oz-eq.	7.5-8 oz-eq.
Milk	2-3 c.	3 c.	3 c.	3 c.	3 c.	3 c.	3 c.	3 c.
Healthy Oils	4 tsp.	5 tsp.	5 tsp.	6 tsp.	6 tsp.	7 tsp.	8 tsp.	8 tsp.

Day/Date: _____

Breakfast: _____ Lunch: _____

Dinner: _____ Snack: _____

Group	Fruits	Vegetables	Grains	Meat & Beans	Milk	Oils
Goal Amount						
Estimate Your Total						
Increase ⇧ or Decrease? ⇩						

Physical Activity: _____ Spiritual Activity: _____

Steps/Miles/Minutes: _____

Day/Date: _____

Breakfast: _____ Lunch: _____

Dinner: _____ Snack: _____

Group	Fruits	Vegetables	Grains	Meat & Beans	Milk	Oils
Goal Amount						
Estimate Your Total						
Increase ⇧ or Decrease? ⇩						

Physical Activity: _____ Spiritual Activity: _____

Steps/Miles/Minutes: _____

Day/Date: _____

Breakfast: _____ Lunch: _____

Dinner: _____ Snack: _____

Group	Fruits	Vegetables	Grains	Meat & Beans	Milk	Oils
Goal Amount						
Estimate Your Total						
Increase ⇧ or Decrease? ⇩						

Physical Activity: _____ Spiritual Activity: _____

Steps/Miles/Minutes: _____

Day/Date: _____

Breakfast: _____ Lunch: _____

Dinner: _____ Snack: _____

Group	Fruits	Vegetables	Grains	Meat & Beans	Milk	Oils
Goal Amount						
Estimate Your Total						
Increase ⇧ or Decrease? ⇩						

Physical Activity: _____ Spiritual Activity: _____

Steps/Miles/Minutes: _____ _____

Day/Date: _____

Breakfast: _____ Lunch: _____

Dinner: _____ Snack: _____

Group	Fruits	Vegetables	Grains	Meat & Beans	Milk	Oils
Goal Amount						
Estimate Your Total						
Increase ⇧ or Decrease? ⇩						

Physical Activity: _____ Spiritual Activity: _____

Steps/Miles/Minutes: _____ _____

Day/Date: _____

Breakfast: _____ Lunch: _____

Dinner: _____ Snack: _____

Group	Fruits	Vegetables	Grains	Meat & Beans	Milk	Oils
Goal Amount						
Estimate Your Total						
Increase ⇧ or Decrease? ⇩						

Physical Activity: _____ Spiritual Activity: _____

Steps/Miles/Minutes: _____ _____

Day/Date: _____

Breakfast: _____ Lunch: _____

Dinner: _____ Snack: _____

Group	Fruits	Vegetables	Grains	Meat & Beans	Milk	Oils
Goal Amount						
Estimate Your Total						
Increase ⇧ or Decrease? ⇩						

Physical Activity: _____ Spiritual Activity: _____

Steps/Miles/Minutes: _____ _____

Live It Tracker

Name: _____ Loss/gain: _____ lbs.

Date: _____ Week #: _____ Calorie Range: _____ My food goal for next week: _____

Activity Level: None, < 30 min/day, 30-60 min/day, 60+ min/day My activity goal for next week: _____

Group	Daily Calories							
	1300-1400	1500-1600	1700-1800	1900-2000	2100-2200	2300-2400	2500-2600	2700-2800
Fruits	1.5-2 c.	1.5-2 c.	1.5-2 c.	2-2.5 c.	2-2.5 c.	2.5-3.5 c.	3.5-4.5 c.	3.5-4.5 c.
Vegetables	1.5-2 c.	2-2.5 c.	2.5-3 c.	2.5-3 c.	3-3.5 c.	3.5-4.5 c.	4.5-5 c.	4.5-5 c.
Grains	5 oz-eq.	5-6 oz-eq.	6-7 oz-eq.	6-7 oz-eq.	7-8 oz-eq.	8-9 oz-eq.	9-10 oz-eq.	10-11 oz-eq.
Meat & Beans	4 oz-eq.	5 oz-eq.	5-5.5 oz-eq.	5.5-6.5 oz-eq.	6.5-7 oz-eq.	7-7.5 oz-eq.	7-7.5 oz-eq.	7.5-8 oz-eq.
Milk	2-3 c.	3 c.	3 c.	3 c.	3 c.	3 c.	3 c.	3 c.
Healthy Oils	4 tsp.	5 tsp.	5 tsp.	6 tsp.	6 tsp.	7 tsp.	8 tsp.	8 tsp.

Day/Date: _____

Breakfast: _____   Lunch: _____

Dinner: _____   Snack: _____

Group	Fruits	Vegetables	Grains	Meat & Beans	Milk	Oils
Goal Amount						
Estimate Your Total						
Increase ⇧ or Decrease? ⇩						

Physical Activity: _____   Spiritual Activity: _____

Steps/Miles/Minutes: _____

Day/Date: _____

Breakfast: _____   Lunch: _____

Dinner: _____   Snack: _____

Group	Fruits	Vegetables	Grains	Meat & Beans	Milk	Oils
Goal Amount						
Estimate Your Total						
Increase ⇧ or Decrease? ⇩						

Physical Activity: _____   Spiritual Activity: _____

Steps/Miles/Minutes: _____

Day/Date: _____

Breakfast: _____   Lunch: _____

Dinner: _____   Snack: _____

Group	Fruits	Vegetables	Grains	Meat & Beans	Milk	Oils
Goal Amount						
Estimate Your Total						
Increase ⇧ or Decrease? ⇩						

Physical Activity: _____   Spiritual Activity: _____

Steps/Miles/Minutes: _____

Day/Date: _____

Breakfast: _____ Lunch: _____

Dinner: _____ Snack: _____
_____ _____

Group	Fruits	Vegetables	Grains	Meat & Beans	Milk	Oils
Goal Amount						
Estimate Your Total						
Increase ⇧ or Decrease? ⇩						

Physical Activity: _____ Spiritual Activity: _____

Steps/Miles/Minutes: _____ _____

Day/Date: _____

Breakfast: _____ Lunch: _____

Dinner: _____ Snack: _____
_____ _____

Group	Fruits	Vegetables	Grains	Meat & Beans	Milk	Oils
Goal Amount						
Estimate Your Total						
Increase ⇧ or Decrease? ⇩						

Physical Activity: _____ Spiritual Activity: _____

Steps/Miles/Minutes: _____ _____

Day/Date: _____

Breakfast: _____ Lunch: _____

Dinner: _____ Snack: _____
_____ _____

Group	Fruits	Vegetables	Grains	Meat & Beans	Milk	Oils
Goal Amount						
Estimate Your Total						
Increase ⇧ or Decrease? ⇩						

Physical Activity: _____ Spiritual Activity: _____

Steps/Miles/Minutes: _____ _____

Day/Date: _____

Breakfast: _____ Lunch: _____

Dinner: _____ Snack: _____
_____ _____

Group	Fruits	Vegetables	Grains	Meat & Beans	Milk	Oils
Goal Amount						
Estimate Your Total						
Increase ⇧ or Decrease? ⇩						

Physical Activity: _____ Spiritual Activity: _____

Steps/Miles/Minutes: _____ _____

Live It Tracker

Name: _____ Loss/gain: _____ lbs.

Date: _____ Week #: ____ Calorie Range: _____ My food goal for next week: _____

Activity Level: None, < 30 min/day, 30-60 min/day, 60+ min/day   My activity goal for next week: _____

Group	Daily Calories							
	1300-1400	1500-1600	1700-1800	1900-2000	2100-2200	2300-2400	2500-2600	2700-2800
Fruits	1.5-2 c.	1.5-2 c.	1.5-2 c.	2-2.5 c.	2-2.5 c.	2.5-3.5 c.	3.5-4.5 c.	3.5-4.5 c.
Vegetables	1.5-2 c.	2-2.5 c.	2.5-3 c.	2.5-3 c.	3-3.5 c.	3.5-4.5 c.	4.5-5 c.	4.5-5 c.
Grains	5 oz-eq.	5-6 oz-eq.	6-7 oz-eq.	6-7 oz-eq.	7-8 oz-eq.	8-9 oz-eq.	9-10 oz-eq.	10-11 oz-eq.
Meat & Beans	4 oz-eq.	5 oz-eq.	5-5.5 oz-eq.	5.5-6.5 oz-eq.	6.5-7 oz-eq.	7-7.5 oz-eq.	7-7.5 oz-eq.	7.5-8 oz-eq.
Milk	2-3 c.	3 c.	3 c.	3 c.	3 c.	3 c.	3 c.	3 c.
Healthy Oils	4 tsp.	5 tsp.	5 tsp.	6 tsp.	6 tsp.	7 tsp.	8 tsp.	8 tsp.

Day/Date:

Breakfast: _____ Lunch: _____

Dinner: _____ Snack: _____

Group	Fruits	Vegetables	Grains	Meat & Beans	Milk	Oils
Goal Amount						
Estimate Your Total						
Increase ⇧ or Decrease? ⇩						

Physical Activity: _____ Spiritual Activity: _____

Steps/Miles/Minutes: _____

Day/Date:

Breakfast: _____ Lunch: _____

Dinner: _____ Snack: _____

Group	Fruits	Vegetables	Grains	Meat & Beans	Milk	Oils
Goal Amount						
Estimate Your Total						
Increase ⇧ or Decrease? ⇩						

Physical Activity: _____ Spiritual Activity: _____

Steps/Miles/Minutes: _____

Day/Date:

Breakfast: _____ Lunch: _____

Dinner: _____ Snack: _____

Group	Fruits	Vegetables	Grains	Meat & Beans	Milk	Oils
Goal Amount						
Estimate Your Total						
Increase ⇧ or Decrease? ⇩						

Physical Activity: _____ Spiritual Activity: _____

Steps/Miles/Minutes: _____

Day/Date: _____

Breakfast: _____   Lunch: _____
_____

Dinner: _____   Snack: _____
_____

Group	Fruits	Vegetables	Grains	Meat & Beans	Milk	Oils
Goal Amount						
Estimate Your Total						
Increase ⇧ or Decrease? ⇩						

Physical Activity: _____   Spiritual Activity: _____
Steps/Miles/Minutes: _____   _____

Day/Date: _____

Breakfast: _____   Lunch: _____
_____

Dinner: _____   Snack: _____
_____

Group	Fruits	Vegetables	Grains	Meat & Beans	Milk	Oils
Goal Amount						
Estimate Your Total						
Increase ⇧ or Decrease? ⇩						

Physical Activity: _____   Spiritual Activity: _____
Steps/Miles/Minutes: _____   _____

Day/Date: _____

Breakfast: _____   Lunch: _____
_____

Dinner: _____   Snack: _____
_____

Group	Fruits	Vegetables	Grains	Meat & Beans	Milk	Oils
Goal Amount						
Estimate Your Total						
Increase ⇧ or Decrease? ⇩						

Physical Activity: _____   Spiritual Activity: _____
Steps/Miles/Minutes: _____   _____

Day/Date: _____

Breakfast: _____   Lunch: _____
_____

Dinner: _____   Snack: _____
_____

Group	Fruits	Vegetables	Grains	Meat & Beans	Milk	Oils
Goal Amount						
Estimate Your Total						
Increase ⇧ or Decrease? ⇩						

Physical Activity: _____   Spiritual Activity: _____
Steps/Miles/Minutes: _____   _____

Live It Tracker

Name: _____ Loss/gain: _____ lbs.

Date: _____ Week #: _____ Calorie Range: _____ My food goal for next week: _____

Activity Level: None, < 30 min/day, 30-60 min/day, 60+ min/day   My activity goal for next week: _____

Group	Daily Calories							
	1300-1400	1500-1600	1700-1800	1900-2000	2100-2200	2300-2400	2500-2600	2700-2800
Fruits	1.5-2 c.	1.5-2 c.	1.5-2 c.	2-2.5 c.	2-2.5 c.	2.5-3.5 c.	3.5-4.5 c.	3.5-4.5 c.
Vegetables	1.5-2 c.	2-2.5 c.	2.5-3 c.	2.5-3 c.	3-3.5 c.	3.5-4.5 c.	4.5-5 c.	4.5-5 c.
Grains	5 oz-eq.	5-6 oz-eq.	6-7 oz-eq.	6-7 oz-eq.	7-8 oz-eq.	8-9 oz-eq.	9-10 oz-eq.	10-11 oz-eq.
Meat & Beans	4 oz-eq.	5 oz-eq.	5-5.5 oz-eq.	5.5-6.5 oz-eq.	6.5-7 oz-eq.	7-7.5 oz-eq.	7-7.5 oz-eq.	7.5-8 oz-eq.
Milk	2-3 c.	3 c.	3 c.	3 c.	3 c.	3 c.	3 c.	3 c.
Healthy Oils	4 tsp.	5 tsp.	5 tsp.	6 tsp.	6 tsp.	7 tsp.	8 tsp.	8 tsp.

Day/Date: _____

Breakfast: _____ Lunch: _____

Dinner: _____ Snack: _____

Group	Fruits	Vegetables	Grains	Meat & Beans	Milk	Oils
Goal Amount						
Estimate Your Total						
Increase ⬆ or Decrease? ⬇						

Physical Activity: _____ Spiritual Activity: _____

Steps/Miles/Minutes: _____

Day/Date: _____

Breakfast: _____ Lunch: _____

Dinner: _____ Snack: _____

Group	Fruits	Vegetables	Grains	Meat & Beans	Milk	Oils
Goal Amount						
Estimate Your Total						
Increase ⬆ or Decrease? ⬇						

Physical Activity: _____ Spiritual Activity: _____

Steps/Miles/Minutes: _____

Day/Date: _____

Breakfast: _____ Lunch: _____

Dinner: _____ Snack: _____

Group	Fruits	Vegetables	Grains	Meat & Beans	Milk	Oils
Goal Amount						
Estimate Your Total						
Increase ⬆ or Decrease? ⬇						

Physical Activity: _____ Spiritual Activity: _____

Steps/Miles/Minutes: _____

Day/Date: _____

Breakfast: _____ Lunch: _____

Dinner: _____ Snack: _____

Group	Fruits	Vegetables	Grains	Meat & Beans	Milk	Oils
Goal Amount						
Estimate Your Total						
Increase ⇧ or Decrease? ⇩						

Physical Activity: _____ Spiritual Activity: _____

Steps/Miles/Minutes: _____

Day/Date: _____

Breakfast: _____ Lunch: _____

Dinner: _____ Snack: _____

Group	Fruits	Vegetables	Grains	Meat & Beans	Milk	Oils
Goal Amount						
Estimate Your Total						
Increase ⇧ or Decrease? ⇩						

Physical Activity: _____ Spiritual Activity: _____

Steps/Miles/Minutes: _____

Day/Date: _____

Breakfast: _____ Lunch: _____

Dinner: _____ Snack: _____

Group	Fruits	Vegetables	Grains	Meat & Beans	Milk	Oils
Goal Amount						
Estimate Your Total						
Increase ⇧ or Decrease? ⇩						

Physical Activity: _____ Spiritual Activity: _____

Steps/Miles/Minutes: _____

Day/Date: _____

Breakfast: _____ Lunch: _____

Dinner: _____ Snack: _____

Group	Fruits	Vegetables	Grains	Meat & Beans	Milk	Oils
Goal Amount						
Estimate Your Total						
Increase ⇧ or Decrease? ⇩						

Physical Activity: _____ Spiritual Activity: _____

Steps/Miles/Minutes: _____

Live It Tracker

Name: _____ Loss/gain: _____ lbs.

Date: _____ Week #: _____ Calorie Range: _____ My food goal for next week: _____

Activity Level: None, < 30 min/day, 30-60 min/day, 60+ min/day My activity goal for next week: _____

Group	Daily Calories							
	1300-1400	1500-1600	1700-1800	1900-2000	2100-2200	2300-2400	2500-2600	2700-2800
Fruits	1.5-2 c.	1.5-2 c.	1.5-2 c.	2-2.5 c.	2-2.5 c.	2.5-3.5 c.	3.5-4.5 c.	3.5-4.5 c.
Vegetables	1.5-2 c.	2-2.5 c.	2.5-3 c.	2.5-3 c.	3-3.5 c.	3.5-4.5 c.	4.5-5 c.	4.5-5 c.
Grains	5 oz-eq.	5-6 oz-eq.	6-7 oz-eq.	6-7 oz-eq.	7-8 oz-eq.	8-9 oz-eq.	9-10 oz-eq.	10-11 oz-eq.
Meat & Beans	4 oz-eq.	5 oz-eq.	5-5.5 oz-eq.	5.5-6.5 oz-eq.	6.5-7 oz-eq.	7-7.5 oz-eq.	7-7.5 oz-eq.	7.5-8 oz-eq.
Milk	2-3 c.	3 c.	3 c.	3 c.	3 c.	3 c.	3 c.	3 c.
Healthy Oils	4 tsp.	5 tsp.	5 tsp.	6 tsp.	6 tsp.	7 tsp.	8 tsp.	8 tsp.

Day/Date: _____

Breakfast: _____ Lunch: _____

Dinner: _____ Snack: _____

Group	Fruits	Vegetables	Grains	Meat & Beans	Milk	Oils
Goal Amount						
Estimate Your Total						
Increase ⇧ or Decrease? ⇩						

Physical Activity: _____ Spiritual Activity: _____

Steps/Miles/Minutes: _____

Day/Date: _____

Breakfast: _____ Lunch: _____

Dinner: _____ Snack: _____

Group	Fruits	Vegetables	Grains	Meat & Beans	Milk	Oils
Goal Amount						
Estimate Your Total						
Increase ⇧ or Decrease? ⇩						

Physical Activity: _____ Spiritual Activity: _____

Steps/Miles/Minutes: _____

Day/Date: _____

Breakfast: _____ Lunch: _____

Dinner: _____ Snack: _____

Group	Fruits	Vegetables	Grains	Meat & Beans	Milk	Oils
Goal Amount						
Estimate Your Total						
Increase ⇧ or Decrease? ⇩						

Physical Activity: _____ Spiritual Activity: _____

Steps/Miles/Minutes: _____

Day/Date: _____

Breakfast: _____ Lunch: _____

Dinner: _____ Snack: _____

Group	Fruits	Vegetables	Grains	Meat & Beans	Milk	Oils
Goal Amount						
Estimate Your Total						
Increase ⇧ or Decrease? ⇩						

Physical Activity: _____ Spiritual Activity: _____

Steps/Miles/Minutes: _____

Day/Date: _____

Breakfast: _____ Lunch: _____

Dinner: _____ Snack: _____

Group	Fruits	Vegetables	Grains	Meat & Beans	Milk	Oils
Goal Amount						
Estimate Your Total						
Increase ⇧ or Decrease? ⇩						

Physical Activity: _____ Spiritual Activity: _____

Steps/Miles/Minutes: _____

Day/Date: _____

Breakfast: _____ Lunch: _____

Dinner: _____ Snack: _____

Group	Fruits	Vegetables	Grains	Meat & Beans	Milk	Oils
Goal Amount						
Estimate Your Total						
Increase ⇧ or Decrease? ⇩						

Physical Activity: _____ Spiritual Activity: _____

Steps/Miles/Minutes: _____

Day/Date: _____

Breakfast: _____ Lunch: _____

Dinner: _____ Snack: _____

Group	Fruits	Vegetables	Grains	Meat & Beans	Milk	Oils
Goal Amount						
Estimate Your Total						
Increase ⇧ or Decrease? ⇩						

Physical Activity: _____ Spiritual Activity: _____

Steps/Miles/Minutes: _____

Live It Tracker

Name: _____ Loss/gain: _____ lbs.

Date: _____ Week #: _____ Calorie Range: _____ My food goal for next week: _____

Activity Level: None, < 30 min/day, 30-60 min/day, 60+ min/day My activity goal for next week: _____

Group	Daily Calories							
	1300-1400	1500-1600	1700-1800	1900-2000	2100-2200	2300-2400	2500-2600	2700-2800
Fruits	1.5-2 c.	1.5-2 c.	1.5-2 c.	2-2.5 c.	2-2.5 c.	2.5-3.5 c.	3.5-4.5 c.	3.5-4.5 c.
Vegetables	1.5-2 c.	2-2.5 c.	2.5-3 c.	2.5-3 c.	3-3.5 c.	3.5-4.5 c.	4.5-5 c.	4.5-5 c.
Grains	5 oz-eq.	5-6 oz-eq.	6-7 oz-eq.	6-7 oz-eq.	7-8 oz-eq.	8-9 oz-eq.	9-10 oz-eq.	10-11 oz-eq.
Meat & Beans	4 oz-eq.	5 oz-eq.	5-5.5 oz-eq.	5.5-6.5 oz-eq.	6.5-7 oz-eq.	7-7.5 oz-eq.	7-7.5 oz-eq.	7.5-8 oz-eq.
Milk	2-3 c.	3 c.	3 c.	3 c.	3 c.	3 c.	3 c.	3 c.
Healthy Oils	4 tsp.	5 tsp.	5 tsp.	6 tsp.	6 tsp.	7 tsp.	8 tsp.	8 tsp.

Day/Date: _____

Breakfast: _____ Lunch: _____

Dinner: _____ Snack: _____

Group	Fruits	Vegetables	Grains	Meat & Beans	Milk	Oils
Goal Amount						
Estimate Your Total						
Increase ⇧ or Decrease? ⇩						

Physical Activity: _____ Spiritual Activity: _____

Steps/Miles/Minutes: _____

Day/Date: _____

Breakfast: _____ Lunch: _____

Dinner: _____ Snack: _____

Group	Fruits	Vegetables	Grains	Meat & Beans	Milk	Oils
Goal Amount						
Estimate Your Total						
Increase ⇧ or Decrease? ⇩						

Physical Activity: _____ Spiritual Activity: _____

Steps/Miles/Minutes: _____

Day/Date: _____

Breakfast: _____ Lunch: _____

Dinner: _____ Snack: _____

Group	Fruits	Vegetables	Grains	Meat & Beans	Milk	Oils
Goal Amount						
Estimate Your Total						
Increase ⇧ or Decrease? ⇩						

Physical Activity: _____ Spiritual Activity: _____

Steps/Miles/Minutes: _____

Day/Date: _____

Breakfast: _____   Lunch: _____

Dinner: _____   Snack: _____

Group	Fruits	Vegetables	Grains	Meat & Beans	Milk	Oils
Goal Amount						
Estimate Your Total						
Increase ⇧ or Decrease? ⇩						

Physical Activity: _____   Spiritual Activity: _____

Steps/Miles/Minutes: _____   _____

Day/Date: _____

Breakfast: _____   Lunch: _____

Dinner: _____   Snack: _____

Group	Fruits	Vegetables	Grains	Meat & Beans	Milk	Oils
Goal Amount						
Estimate Your Total						
Increase ⇧ or Decrease? ⇩						

Physical Activity: _____   Spiritual Activity: _____

Steps/Miles/Minutes: _____   _____

Day/Date: _____

Breakfast: _____   Lunch: _____

Dinner: _____   Snack: _____

Group	Fruits	Vegetables	Grains	Meat & Beans	Milk	Oils
Goal Amount						
Estimate Your Total						
Increase ⇧ or Decrease? ⇩						

Physical Activity: _____   Spiritual Activity: _____

Steps/Miles/Minutes: _____   _____

Day/Date: _____

Breakfast: _____   Lunch: _____

Dinner: _____   Snack: _____

Group	Fruits	Vegetables	Grains	Meat & Beans	Milk	Oils
Goal Amount						
Estimate Your Total						
Increase ⇧ or Decrease? ⇩						

Physical Activity: _____   Spiritual Activity: _____

Steps/Miles/Minutes: _____   _____

Live It Tracker

Name: _____ Loss/gain: _____ lbs.

Date: _____ Week #: _____ Calorie Range: _____ My food goal for next week: _____

Activity Level: None, < 30 min/day, 30-60 min/day, 60+ min/day My activity goal for next week: _____

Group	Daily Calories							
	1300-1400	1500-1600	1700-1800	1900-2000	2100-2200	2300-2400	2500-2600	2700-2800
Fruits	1.5-2 c.	1.5-2 c.	1.5-2 c.	2-2.5 c.	2-2.5 c.	2.5-3.5 c.	3.5-4.5 c.	3.5-4.5 c.
Vegetables	1.5-2 c.	2-2.5 c.	2.5-3 c.	2.5-3 c.	3-3.5 c.	3.5-4.5 c.	4.5-5 c.	4.5-5 c.
Grains	5 oz-eq.	5-6 oz-eq.	6-7 oz-eq.	6-7 oz-eq.	7-8 oz-eq.	8-9 oz-eq.	9-10 oz-eq.	10-11 oz-eq.
Meat & Beans	4 oz-eq.	5 oz-eq.	5-5.5 oz-eq.	5.5-6.5 oz-eq.	6.5-7 oz-eq.	7-7.5 oz-eq.	7-7.5 oz-eq.	7.5-8 oz-eq.
Milk	2-3 c.	3 c.	3 c.	3 c.	3 c.	3 c.	3 c.	3 c.
Healthy Oils	4 tsp.	5 tsp.	5 tsp.	6 tsp.	6 tsp.	7 tsp.	8 tsp.	8 tsp.

Day/Date: _____

Breakfast: _____ Lunch: _____

Dinner: _____ Snack: _____

Group	Fruits	Vegetables	Grains	Meat & Beans	Milk	Oils
Goal Amount						
Estimate Your Total						
Increase ⇧ or Decrease? ⇩						

Physical Activity: _____ Spiritual Activity: _____

Steps/Miles/Minutes: _____ _____

Day/Date: _____

Breakfast: _____ Lunch: _____

Dinner: _____ Snack: _____

Group	Fruits	Vegetables	Grains	Meat & Beans	Milk	Oils
Goal Amount						
Estimate Your Total						
Increase ⇧ or Decrease? ⇩						

Physical Activity: _____ Spiritual Activity: _____

Steps/Miles/Minutes: _____ _____

Day/Date: _____

Breakfast: _____ Lunch: _____

Dinner: _____ Snack: _____

Group	Fruits	Vegetables	Grains	Meat & Beans	Milk	Oils
Goal Amount						
Estimate Your Total						
Increase ⇧ or Decrease? ⇩						

Physical Activity: _____ Spiritual Activity: _____

Steps/Miles/Minutes: _____ _____

Day/Date: ___

Breakfast: _____ Lunch: _____

Dinner: _____ Snack: _____

Group	Fruits	Vegetables	Grains	Meat & Beans	Milk	Oils
Goal Amount						
Estimate Your Total						
Increase ⬆ or Decrease? ⬇						

Physical Activity: _____ Spiritual Activity: _____

Steps/Miles/Minutes: _____

Day/Date: ___

Breakfast: _____ Lunch: _____

Dinner: _____ Snack: _____

Group	Fruits	Vegetables	Grains	Meat & Beans	Milk	Oils
Goal Amount						
Estimate Your Total						
Increase ⬆ or Decrease? ⬇						

Physical Activity: _____ Spiritual Activity: _____

Steps/Miles/Minutes: _____

Day/Date: ___

Breakfast: _____ Lunch: _____

Dinner: _____ Snack: _____

Group	Fruits	Vegetables	Grains	Meat & Beans	Milk	Oils
Goal Amount						
Estimate Your Total						
Increase ⬆ or Decrease? ⬇						

Physical Activity: _____ Spiritual Activity: _____

Steps/Miles/Minutes: _____

Day/Date: ___

Breakfast: _____ Lunch: _____

Dinner: _____ Snack: _____

Group	Fruits	Vegetables	Grains	Meat & Beans	Milk	Oils
Goal Amount						
Estimate Your Total						
Increase ⬆ or Decrease? ⬇						

Physical Activity: _____ Spiritual Activity: _____

Steps/Miles/Minutes: _____

let's count our miles!

Join the 100-Mile Club this Session

Can't walk that mile yet? Don't be discouraged! There are exercises you can do to strengthen your body and burn those extra calories. Keep a record on your Live It Tracker of the number of minutes you do these common physical activities, convert those minutes to miles following the chart below, and then mark off each mile you have completed on the chart found on the back of the back cover. Report your miles to your 100-Mile Club representative when you first arrive each week. Remember, you are not competing with anyone else . . . just yourself. Your job is to strive reach 100 miles before the last meeting in this session. You can do it—just keep on moving!

Walking

slowly, 2 mph	30 min. = 156 cal. = 1 mile
moderately, 3 mph	20 min. = 156 cal. = 1 mile
very briskly, 4 mph	15 min. = 156 cal. = 1 mile
speed walking	10 min. = 156 cal. = 1 mile
up stairs	13 min. = 159 cal. = 1 mile

Running/Jogging

10 min. = 156 cal. = 1 mile

Cycling Outdoors

slowly, <10 mph	20 min. = 156 cal. = 1 mile
light effort, 10-12 mph	12 min. = 156 cal. = 1 mile
moderate effort, 12-14 mph.	10 min. = 156 cal. = 1 mile
vigorous effort, 14-16 mph	7.5 min. = 156 cal. = 1 mile
very fast, 16-19 mph	6.5 min. = 152 cal. = 1 mile

Sports Activities

Playing tennis (singles)	10 min. = 156 cal. = 1 mile
Swimming	
light to moderate effort	11 min. = 152 cal. = 1 mile
fast, vigorous effort	7.5 min. = 156 cal. = 1 mile
Softball	15 min. = 156 cal. = 1 mile
Golf	20 min. = 156 cal = 1 mile
Rollerblading	6.5 min. = 152 cal. = 1 mile
Ice skating	11 min. = 152 cal. = 1 mile

Jumping rope	7.5 min. = 156 cal. = 1 mile
Basketball	12 min. = 156 cal. = 1 mile
Soccer (casual)	15 min. = 159 cal. = 1 mile

Around the House

Mowing grass	22 min. = 156 cal. = 1 mile
Mopping, sweeping, vacuuming	19.5 min. = 155 cal. = 1 mile
Cooking	40 min. =160 cal. = 1 mile
Gardening	19 min. = 156 cal. = 1 mile
Housework (general)	35 min. = 156 cal. = 1 mile
Ironing	45 min. = 153 cal. = 1 mile
Raking leaves	25 min. = 150 cal. = 1 mile
Washing car	23 min. = 156 cal. = 1 mile
Washing dishes	45 min. = 153 cal. = 1 mile

At the Gym

Stair machine	8.5 min. = 155 cal. = 1 mile
Stationary bike	
slowly, 10 mph	30 min. = 156 cal. = 1 mile
moderately, 10-13 mph	15 min. = 156 cal. = 1 mile
vigorously, 13-16 mph	7.5 min. = 156 cal. = 1 mile
briskly, 16-19 mph	6.5 min. = 156 cal. = 1 mile
Elliptical trainer	12 min. = 156 cal. = 1 mile
Weight machines (used vigorously)	13 min. = 152 cal.=1 mile
Aerobics	
low impact	15 min. = 156 cal. = 1 mile
high impact	12 min. = 156 cal. = 1 mile
water	20 min. = 156 cal. = 1 mile
Pilates	15 min. = 156 cal. = 1 mile
Raquetball (casual)	15 min. = 159 cal. = 1 mile
Stretching exercises	25 min. = 150 cal. = 1 mile
Weight lifting (also works for weight	
machines used moderately or gently)	30 min. = 156 cal. = 1 mile

Family Leisure

Playing piano	37 min. = 155 cal. = 1 mile
Jumping rope	10 min. = 152 cal. = 1 mile
Skating (moderate)	20 min. = 152 cal. = 1 mile
Swimming	
moderate	17 min. = 156 cal. = 1 mile
vigorous	10 min. = 148 cal. = 1 mile
Table tennis	25 min. = 150 cal. = 1 mile
Walk/run/play with kids	25 min. = 150 cal. = 1 mile